Current Therapy of Communication Disorders

DYSARTHRIA AND APRAXIA

Other volumes in the series:

Current Therapy of Communication Disorders

DYSARTHRIA AND APRAXIA

edited by
William H. Perkins, Ph.D.
University of Southern California

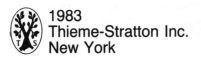 1983
Thieme-Stratton Inc.
New York

Georg Thieme Verlag
Stuttgart • New York

Acknowledgment
I am grateful to James Aten, Ray Kent, Jeri Logemann, and
John Rosenbek for their guidance in the selection of therapies
and authors for this volume.

Publisher: Thieme-Stratton Inc.
381 Park Avenue South
New York, New York

Cover typography by M. Losaw

Printed in the United States of America

CURRENT THERAPY OF COMMUNICATION
DISORDERS
Dysarthria and Apraxia
edited by William H. Perkins

TMP ISBN 0-86577-404-8 (pbk)

Contents

Contributing Authors

James L. Aten, Ph.D.
Veterans Administration Medical Center
Long Beach, CA

Bill Berry, Ph.D.
Veterans Administration Medical Center
Memphis, TN

David R. Beukelman, Ph.D.
University of Washington, Seattle, WA

Robert W. Blakeley, Ph.D.
University of Oregon, Portland, OR

Craig W. Linebaugh, Ph.D.
The George Washington University, Washington, D.C.

Judy K. Montgomery, M.A.
Fountain Valley School District, Fountain Valley, CA

Thomas Murry, Ph.D.
Veterans Administration Medical Center, San Diego,
CA

Edward D. Mysak, Ph.D.
Teachers College, Columbia University,
New York, NY

John C. Rosenbek, Ph.D.
Wm. S. Middleton Memorial Veterans Administration
Hospital, Madison, WI

Franklin H. Silverman, Ph.D.
Marquette University, Milwaukee, WI

FOREWORD TO THE SERIES

Roughly a billion dollars is invested annually in the clinical service of speech, language, and hearing disorders. Were this service provided to only one person, our best effort would be mandatory. The magnitude of the investment merely heightens the importance of our clinical responsibility.

The volumes in this *Current Therapy* series are an effort to help meet this responsibility. They are intended for the practicing clinician who needs a convenient reference for therapy of any problem of speech, language, or hearing. Each volume contains as many chapters as were required to present all of the forms of therapy which are currently differentiated for disorders of language, articulation, voice, fluency, and hearing in children and adults. One could call this a "distinctive feature" approach in the sense that therapy of any disorder that is distinguished from therapy of another disorder by at least one feature of treatment warranted a separate chapter.

To avoid repeating general procedures for learning new responses, transferring them to daily life, and making them permanent, they are presented in the volume, *General Principles of Therapy*. Each general technique is described from the standpoint of whatever theory of learning it is mainly derived. For example, response shaping is presented as an operant procedure, modeling as a procedure of cognitive learning theory.

These procedures are not described systematically in the other volumes. Instead, each chapter in these volumes is a free standing, terse, procedural account of a specific therapy as practiced by the author for a specific type of disorder.

The focus of each volume is exclusively on treatment. Matters of assessment, diagnosis, and rationale are included only to the extent that they are needed to clarify characteristics of the person for whom the therapy is intended, and the reasons for it. Credibility of the therapy is embedded in the credibility of the authors, who were selected on the best advice I could obtain. Asking authors to describe what they do was tantamount to asking them to evaluate our entire treatment-research literature. Because they must make the most responsible judgment they can for each person they serve, their treatment recognizes the research that has therapy value and goes beyond science to include the intangible verities of clinical practice as an art.

William H. Perkins
Editor

PREFACE

My efforts to organize therapies of dysarthria and apraxia have a checkered history. Originally, I thought a behavioral organization would be sensibly consistent with the purpose of the series. After all, a compendium of therapies of communication disorders is necessarily about modification of speech and language performance. Even though dysarthria and apraxia are manifestations of neuropathology, medical and surgical procedures are not among the treatment techniques of the speech-language pathologist or audiologist. The learning process is our sole clinical tool, and language, articulation, voice, and fluency are the tools of communicative behavior to which we apply this tool. What could be more sensible, I reasoned, than to classify therapies of dysarthria and apraxia under the types of speaking behavior affected? Thus, dysarthria ended up under both voice and articulation; apraxia was under fluency.

The illogic of my logic soon became apparent. The authors I invited were probably as unimpressed with this scheme as readers would eventually have been. At any rate, few authors responded to my invitation. Consultation with clinicians who knew far more about motor speech disorders than I, revealed several important considerations. One was that the prognosis for people with these disorders has an important bearing on realistic goals that can be set for treatment. This determination depends largely on the disease basic to the motor speech disorder. A classification by type of neuropathology would have accommodated a concern for prognosis, but it would have resulted in overlapping and duplicative descriptions of treatment. Although appropriate for medical considerations, classification by disease was considered too inefficient to work well as a basis for describing speech therapy.

The consensus of advice was to retain the classifications of dysarthria that have prevailed in recent years, even though some advisors had reservations about them. The overriding need was to retain the integrity of the person, irrespective of multiplicity of types of impairment he or she might have. This need applied equally to persons with apraxia, and to cerebral-palsied children with their host of disorders, dysarthria being one. Hence, motor speech disorders were accorded a separate volume in which people with each type of disorder could be viewed in terms of the full range of problems that should be considered in their treatment.

William H. Perkins
Editor

PART ONE:
CEREBRAL PALSY
AND DEVELOPMENTAL
APRAXIA

CHAPTER ONE

TREATMENT OF DEVIANT PHONOLOGICAL SYSTEMS: CEREBRAL PALSY

Method of Edward D. Mysak

Cerebral palsy speech disorder reflects an organismic neurological problem that requires an organismic intervention approach. My orientation toward speech habilitation of the cerebral-palsied is reflected in what I call my approach: neurospeech therapy. It is used for patients with any of the major types of cerebral palsy and is applied during childhood, or even during adulthood. Better results are expected, however, when the techniques are applied during the time the central nervous system (CNS) is still in its developmental period. This chapter is confined to a discussion of procedures and techniques designed to improve speech postures and movements in children with cerebral palsy.

PRINCIPLES OF THERAPY

Therapy techniques are based on at least four principles: emergent specificity, reflexization of movement, figure-ground motor stimulation, and integration-elaboration of sensorimotor patterns. Only brief discussions of these principles can be offered here. For more detailed discussions, the reader is referred to appropriate sections of my book on neurospeech therapy (see Selected References).

Emergent Specificity

The principle of emergent specificity is drawn from phylogenetic and ontogenetic concepts related to the development of speech in humans. The principle alerts the clinician to the concepts that speech waits upon (1) the emergence of the individual to the upright posture, which provides the important framework for the speech mechanism, (2) the differentiation of the arms and hands, which allows their use for symbolic gestural and adjunctive gestural behavior, and (3) the

3

freeing of the mouth from crude vegetative activities, which allows its use for speech articulatory movements. In short, and colloquially speaking, the principle reminds the clinician that speech or "mouth talk" gradually emerges from "body," "hands," and "face talk."

Reflexization of Movement

The principle of reflexization of movement is drawn from the relationship between reflexive maturation and motor development; more specifically, the relationship between the development of reflexes and speech postures, and reflexes and speech movements. Accordingly, the emergence of back, elbow, sit, or stand speech postures depends on the integration and elaboration of spinal and brain-stem reflexes by righting reactions and the co-occurring integration of righting reactions by equilibrium reactions. And the emergence of skilled speech breathing, phonation, resonation, and articulation depends on the integration and elaboration of certain protective, emotional, and vegetative reflexes and reflexive vocalization.

I, therefore, do not attempt to develop speech postures directly. Instead, I try to elicit the righting, support, and balance reactions that allow the child to assume and maintain the various postures. Likewise, I do not attempt to develop skilled speech movements directly. Instead, I try to stimulate basic protective, emotional, and vegetative reflexes and their integration as reflected through reflexive voicing and primary talking. More precisely, I work from the premise that speech reflexes form the basic language of the motor speech program.

Figure-Ground Motor Stimulation

The principle of figure-ground motor stimulation is based upon the observation that basic speech postures and basic or skilled speech movements do not develop in strict sequential fashion. For example, during the first 6- to 9-month period in a child's life, one may observe co-developing head balance, sitting, creeping, and assisted standing and walking. With respect to the concept of figure-ground motor activity, however, the sequence of stimulation would be head balance (figure motor pattern) against all other motor patterns (ground motor patterns), then sitting (figure) against the others (ground), then standing against the others and, finally, walking against the others.

The principle of figure-ground motor stimulation is translated into practical therapy procedures by stimulating the range of basic speech postures (e.g., back, elbow, sit, stand speech postures), but with focus on a sequentially appropriate pattern (e.g., sit speech posture) and the range of basic speech movements, but with focus on a sequentially appropriate pattern.

Integration-Elaboration of Sensorimotor Patterns

Integration of sensory inflow may take place at different levels or combinations of levels of integration centers. Therapeutic maneuvers must be designed, therefore, that will stimulate the progressive integration of sensorimotor integration centers by higher ones until the highest possible level of sensorimotor integration has been achieved. A child in the prone position, for example, may not be able to raise the head and support the trunk in the elbow speech posture because of the influence of spinal and brain-stem integration centers manifested by primitive limb-withdrawal patterns and a general increase in flexor tonus. To counteract this manifestation of lower-center integration, I may design a "sensory question" in the form of extending the child's limbs and trunk and outwardly rotating the shoulders, and thereby feeding back stimuli from tactile and proprioceptive receptors that result in a new "motor reply," consisting of upper limb support movements and a head righting and balance reaction. Such a reply implies that the sensory inflow has been rerouted successfully to a higher center of integration.

To facilitate the integration of primitive movement patterns, I use the maneuver of mismatching sensorimotor feedbacks. Integration of a basic movement like the mouth-opening reflex, for example, may be attempted by use of the mismatching maneuver. The maneuver is performed by applying the appropriate stimulus (visual or touch stimuli) and physically resisting the expected response. By denying the lower center the expected sensory feedback, the function of the lower-center may be "unbalanced" and a higher center may be "activated."

To stimulate a new movement pattern, I use the maneuver of matching sensorimotor feedbacks. To stimulate an absent bilabial movement, for example, I provide the sensory feedback associated with the movement by physically bringing the lips into contact (motokinesthetic method). It is hoped that through repetition of such a maneuver the sensory feedback stimulation will excite the corresponding motor feedforward activity.

To stimulate the adjustment of an existing or new movement,

I use the maneuver of correct-response feedback. If, for example, a child attempts to form the /f/ and shows difficulty in making the required labiodental contact, I directly assist so that a more normal contact and, consequently, more normal feedback is provided. I expect that such correct-response feedback maneuvers will lead eventually to correct response performance.

NEUROSPEECH THERAPY

The actual therapy program is divided into two parts: the stimulation of basic movements and the stimulation of skilled movements.

Basic Movements

The stimulation of basic postures and movements or reflexes is fundamental to neurospeech therapy, since it is from basic speech postures and basic listening, hand, and speech movements that skilled speech movements emerge. Table 1 summarizes the program of procedures and techniques used for stimulating basic speech movements.

Preparatory Maneuvers. Therapy is started with three types of preparatory or warm-up maneuvers: pretzeling, reflex conditioning, and body-image formation. Such maneuvers tend to induce physiological relaxation; regularize tone, posture, and movement; and facilitate integration and elaboration of reflexive units.

Pretzeling describes the imposition on the child of irregular postures or "therapeutic discomfort." Resolution of the discomfort occurs when the child moves into more normal postures. For example: with the child in supine position, I may cross the child's legs, or flex one leg under or over the other extended one, or place the hands under the buttocks; with the child in prone position, I may cross one or both of his arms under the chest, or cross the legs in various ways; and with the child in side lying, I may arrange his arms and legs in various and unusual postures. Pretzeling can also be done with the child in the sitting position.

Maneuvers should be executed with a gradual increase in range, direction, and speed, and be routinized so that a program is established and a "workout" is provided that is smooth and rhythmical. Also, I impose the irregular posture to the point where a spontaneous countermovement from the child is elicited—if such a countermovement is not forthcoming I assist or facilitate it. While engaged

Table 1. Summary of Procedures for the Stimulation of Basic Speech Movements

Procedure	Description
Preparatory maneuvers	
Pretzeling	Impose irregular postures in various positions to elicit righting countermovements
Reflex conditioning	Elicit various eye, head, trunk, arm, hand, and leg reflexes to help normalize muscle tone and posture
Supplementary techniques	Use toning and posturing techniques to help regularize muscle tone and body posture
Body-image formation	Use child's hand(s) to delineate body parts and contribute to child's self-concept development
Listening movements	
Protective reflexes	Elicit auditory Moro, eye closing-opening, and mouth-opening reflexes in response to loud, unexpected, unfamiliar sounds
Listening reflexes	Elicit body stilling in response to human vocalization
Tuning reflexes	Elicit changes in respiration and heartbeat in response to various auditory stimuli
Speech postures	
Back patterns	Stimulate movement from prone to back-pattern speech posture (via elemental body-on-body and on-head righting reactions) and balance and support movements (equilibrium reactions in semi-reclining position) to stabilize the posture
Elbow patterns	Stimulate movement from supine to elbow-pattern speech posture (via elemental body-on-body and on-head righting reactions and tuning Landau and chain-in-prone midbrain reactions) and balance and support movements (equilibrium reactions in prone, side lying, and on-forearms) to stabilize the posture
Sit patterns	Stimulate movement from supine to prone, to on-fours, to sit-pattern speech posture (via chain of elemental righting reactions) and balance and support movements (equilibrium reactions in on-fours and in-sitting positions) to stabilize the posture
Stand patterns	Stimulate movement from supine to prone, to on-fours, to on-knees, to half-kneel, to stand speech posture (via chain of elemental righting reactions) and balance and support movements (equilibrium reactions in on-knees, half-kneel, and stand positions) to stabilize the posture
Hand movements	
Protective reflexes	Elicit arm-support and arm-balance reactions in sitting, kneeling, and standing
Progression reflexes	Elicit upper limb movement, upper limb placing, arm walking, and quadrupedal hopping
Vegetative reflexes	Stimulate general hand-to-mouth movements and hand-to-mouth feeding movements
Speech movements	
Protective reflexes	Elicit glottic closing-opening, sneeze-cough, and jaw-jerk and palatal reflexes
Emotional reflexes	Elicit cry, smile, and laugh reflexes
Vegetative reflexes	Stimulate vegetative breathing through inspiratory reflex maneuvers and inspiratory facilitation maneuvers (arm-lift, leg-roll, accordion, butterfly techniques) Facilitate eating movements through 9-factor approach (nursing, positioning, protecting, priming, transporting, grasping, manipulating, preparing, swallowing)
Reflexive vocalization	Encourage movement-associated, hand-to-mouth, and happy-play vocalization

in the routine, I also take every opportunity to name body parts, describe movements, and, in general, converse with the child.

The benefits that may be derived from pretzeling are physiological relaxation through vigorous movement and automatic movement responses resulting from tactile, otolithic, and general proprioceptive stimulation. I also expect improvement in body-part awareness and body-part self-adjustment capacities.

Reflex conditioning usually follows pretzeling and involves the regular elicitation of various reflexes. It is recommended that such conditioning be done at least once a day and that about 20 reflexes be stimulated, each for a number of minutes. I pay special attention to affected limbs and guide them to participate in the expected movements and postures as much as possible. Reflexes are stimulated in accordance with the law of developmental direction as follows: eye, head, trunk, arm, hand, leg, and foot reflexes.

1. Eye reflexes include eye-tracking movements (following finger in all directions and with the child in various postures) and eye-closure reflexes (e.g., McCarthy's).

2. Head reflexes include protective movements (e.g., countermovements in response to the head being moved to various extreme positions), vegetative movements (e.g., rooting), and righting movements (i.e., on-head righting reactions such as the labyrinthine, body, and optical righting reactions).

3. Trunk reflexes include primary sitting, dorsal, and lumbar reflexes and body-on-body righting reactions.

4. Arm reflexes include upper limb movements, arm-support movements, placing reaction of the arm, and arm walking.

5. Hand reflexes include the grasp, finger flexion (e.g., Hoffman's reflex), and Darwinian reflexes (grasp and hang).

6. Leg reflexes include various leg automatisms (i.e., flexion, extension, magnet, cross reflexes), leg support reactions, placing reaction of the leg, primary walking, and hopping reactions.

7. Foot reflexes include ankle clonus and the plantar responses (i.e., flexor and extensor).

8. I also make use of Fay's "unlocking" maneuvers for the hand, arm, and legs, and the Landau, Shaltenbrand, and chain-in-prone reactions. Again, active verbal interaction between client and clinician should accompany reflex conditioning work.

Regular application of reflex conditioning helps prevent tendencies toward fixed postures, maintains and builds muscle volume, allows for physiological relaxation, helps normalize muscle tone and posture, and facilitates volitional movements through simultaneous stimulation of specific reflexes.

Supplementary techniques of at least two types may be used during pretzeling or reflex conditioning maneuvers, and I refer to these as toning and posturing techniques. They are used when pretzeling or eliciting reflexes, if I find that muscle tonus during any one maneuver is too high or too low, or that the child is not able to move into or hold a normal posture.

1. Toning techniques such as quick stroking or tapping of particular muscles, or bouncing the child's buttocks on the floor or on the clinician's knees, may increase tonus, whereas slow rhythmic shaking of a limb or organ, or rocking the child in various directions may decrease tonus.

2. Posturing techniques may be used on the head and trunk, for example. To counter head droop toward the chest, I place one of my extended middle fingers on the forehead and the other on the nape of the neck and guide the head into the normal position. With head droop toward the shoulder, I place one of my middle fingers on the temple and the other on the opposite side of the neck. Accordingly, forward chest droop is counteracted by pressure from one finger on the middle of the sternum and pressure from the other in the lumbar area, and sideways chest droop is adjusted by application of finger pressure on the side of the upper thorax and on the opposite side of the waist. I also use the verbal reinforcers "crooked" and "straight" at the appropriate times.

Body-image formation is the last preparatory maneuver to be used. I expect pretzeling, reflex conditioning, and supplementary techniques to contribute to body-image formation; however, more specific hand-body exploration in conjunction with verbal reinforcement, done in prone, supine, and sit positions, is recommended. In carrying out the maneuvers, I again follow the law of developmental direction. The sequence to follow is head, face, neck, arms, chest, stomach, buttocks, and legs.

Assuming the child is unable to move the hands freely, I guide both together and then one at a time to the various body parts. While the child's hand is in contact with the various body parts, I accompany the hand exploration with running descriptions of the parts.

Since body-image development is integral to sensory-perceptual-symbolic maturation, this preparatory maneuver is an important one.

Listening Movements. I follow the application of the various preparatory maneuvers with techniques for eliciting basic listening movements associated with protective, listening, and tuning reflexes.

Protective reflexes are defined as the extensor startle (auditory Moro reflex), eye-closing (cochleo-palpebral), eye-opening, and mouth-opening reflexes elicited in response to loud, unexpected, or unfamiliar sounds. Since I view the auditory Moro reflex as a stabilizing movement in the prone position, I place the child in prone position and then introduce the unexpected, unfamiliar, or loud sounds. Adaptation to repeated stimuli and replacement of the extensor startle by the flexor startle pattern marks the integration of this early reflex. Since it will be found that closing or opening reflexes of eyes and mouth usually accompany the extensor startle, it is usually unnecessary to stimulate them separately.

Listening reflexes are defined as body stilling (cessation of suckling, for example) in response to human voice. Such passive listening is precursory to active listening (as reflected by "vocal replies" to voiced stimuli), and I recommend its daily stimulation by the use of novel vocalization (done by shifting pitch, loudness, quality, and time factors).

Tuning reflexes are defined as involuntary automatic responses to sound—that is, changes in respiration, heartbeat, and hormonal flow—that tend to enhance listening behavior. I seek to elicit such reflexes (e.g., changes in respiration and heartbeat) through the appropriate choice of stimuli by which to excite listening reflexes.

Regular stimulation of protective, listening, and tuning reflexes contributes to the emergence of skilled listening movements, to be described.

Speech Postures. Depending on the neurophysiological level of the child, I may work on speech postures before listening movements. In order to elicit, establish, and maintain back, elbow, sit, and stand speech postures, certain elemental, tuning, and stabilizing reflexes and reactions are stimulated. I recommend that all four speech postures be stimulated once or twice a day and each movement-to-posture sequence be repeated five to ten times. Depending on the neurophysiological level of the child, stimulation of one or two of the postures over the others may be emphasized. Also, because of space limitations, only the stimulation of the back-pattern speech posture will be described in detail. Procedures for stimulating the other speech postures are similar. Some details for their stimulation may be found by consulting Table 1, and full details may be found by consulting appropriate sections of my book on neurospeech therapy.

Back-pattern speech postures are the first to develop. The primary form is characterized by head in alignment with the body, with head and trunk in a semi-reclining posture, limbs gently flexed and abducted, and hands brought together and to the mouth. Such a posture allows for hand-to-mouth exploration and is conducive to reflexive vocalization. Other forms of the posture include occiput-in-hands, hands-on-crown, hands-on-knees, hands-on-one-knee, and chin-in-hand positions. As is true of all the speech postures identified here, back-pattern speech postures are used throughout life.

The starting position used to stimulate the primary form of the back-pattern speech posture is characterized by the child being in a face-downward position with neck, trunk, and legs extended, right arm in a gently extended posture above the head, and left arm in a flexed push-off position at about the level of the face.

The movement-to-posture sequence used is as follows: I position myself at the child's head and place one hand under the chin and the other at the back of the head. I gently extend and rotate the head until the shoulder girdle, and then the pelvic girdle, follow (body-on-body righting reactions) and, finally, roll-over on the back is accomplished. Once roll-over is accomplished, stimulation of the top of the head with a roll or wedge is recommended to elicit on-head righting in supine and trunk raising to the semi-reclining, back-pattern speech posture. If parts of the movement sequence lag, I physically facilitate the movement. My goal is to facilitate the movement with the least assistance and, finally, without any assistance.

Stabilization of the posture is done through the facilitation of equilibrium reactions in the semi-reclining position. This is done by placing the child's hands on feet, calves, or knees of semiflexed legs, and then I tip the body gently sideways. Two responses are acceptable: a balance reaction, by which the child resists being tipped to the side and rights the body toward the midline, or a support reaction, by which the child reaches out with the limbs and stabilizes the body. If balance and/or support reactions are not forthcoming from the child, I physically facilitate them until they are stimulated.

Elbow-pattern, sit-pattern, and stand-pattern speech postures are similarly stimulated. Each one of the postures has a starting position (same one for elbow, sit, and stand speech postures), a movement-to-posture sequence, and particular stabilization maneuvers.

If it is a physiological given that postural control precedes movement control, then the importance of establishing and maintaining basic speech postures cannot be overstated. We have been remiss in acknowledging the importance of the concept of speech postures and the role of the speech clinician in their development, especially in work with the cerebral-palsied. Basic speech postures provide appropriate background muscle tonus and appropriate background stability for the respiratory-phonatory-resonatory-articulatory complex. Put in motor vehicle terms, in order for the speech motor to run efficiently, it must be mounted in a stable speech chassis.

Hand Movements. At least two forms of "hands talk" may be identified: symbolic gestural and adjunctive gestural. Symbolic gestures include movements such as waving goodbye and reaching out to be picked up, for example; adjunctive gestures include supportive hand movements of a nonspecific nature that usually accompany running speech. Since I believe that hands talk emerges from various types of reflexive hand movements, I simulate such reflexes. I divide these reflexive hand movements into three categories: protective, progression, and vegetative.

Protective reflexes include arm-support and arm-balance movements. I elicit arm-support reactions—that is, limb extension and hand and finger extension toward the side of weight transference in sitting (forward, sideways, and backward) and kneeling positions. I also elicit arm-balance reactions—that is, limb extension and abduction opposite to the side of weight transference in sitting, kneeling, and standing positions.

Progression reflexes include upper limb movement, upper limb placing, arm walking, and quadrupedal hopping. These are stimulated separately if I have not already done so under the reflex conditioning portion of the therapy program.

Vegetative reflexes include hand-to-mouth movements, in general, and hand-to-mouth feeding activity. I usually stimulate both of these activities. Hand-to-mouth activities are stimulated in side lying, supine lying, and sitting positions. With the child in side lying, for example, I place the child in a symmetrical pattern with the shoulders moved forward, and then I bring the hands together and to the mouth. I recommend to parents, and other individuals responsible for feeding, that hand-to-mouth feeding movements should be encouraged by placing the child's hands around the bottle while suckling, and by placing a biscuit in the child's hand and guiding it to the mouth.

As with the concept of speech postures, hands talk also has received too little attention from our field. Its importance to normal speakers should be obvious whenever we observe a lecture, an argument or discussion, or a lively conversation; its importance to handicapped individuals should also be obvious. (Hands talk will be described in the section of the chapter devoted to the stimulation of skilled movements.)

Speech Movements. Certain reflexes that may be called "speech reflexes" form the basic language of the motor speech program and, therefore, should be stimulated daily. These reflexes are basic to feeding movements, later preverbal speech movements, and, finally, to skilled speech movements. They are categorized under protective, emotional, and vegetative reflexes, and reflexive vocalization.

Protective reflexes include glottic closing-opening, sneeze-cough, and jaw-jerk-palatal reflexes. Glottic opening may be stimulated by periodically occluding the child's nostrils by pinching them with the fingers; I sometimes use "aroma therapy" in the form of vinegar or ammonia to elicit reflexive glottic closing. Chemical stimuli, such as soap powder or pepper, or stimulating the nostril area with a wisp of cotton, may trigger sneezing. The sudden introduction of pungent aromas, such as those associated with ammonia, vinegar, and horseradish, may elicit reflexive coughing. I also elicit the jaw jerk (I place the index finger of one hand laterally across the mental prominence of the mandible and briskly tap the finger with the ends of the middle three fingers of my other hand) and the palatal reflex (I elicit velar elevation by touching or stroking the velar raphe with a Q-Tip).

The CNS integration of these reflexes contributes to movements used in voicing and in the production of pressure and mandibular speech sounds.

Emotional reflexes include cry, smile, and laugh reflexes. I recommend that parents, friends, and therapists make efforts to excite smile and laugh behavior daily. Various forms of movements, faces, noises, and touches comprise the appropriate stimuli for smile and laugh behavior. Integration of these reflexes results in their use as speech-tuning reflexes; for example, they may be used to influence vocal color, and speech rate and rhythm.

Vegetative reflexes include those involved with vegetative breathing and those with feeding.

1. Respiration is stimulated by the use of two techniques: inspiratory reflex maneuvers and inspiratory facilitation maneuvers.

a. The inspiratory reflex may be elicited by pressing closed one of the child's nostrils, while the child's mouth is closed, by briefly pressing closed both nostrils or by asking the child to hold the breath for as long as possible, or to breathe out for as long as possible (breath exhaustion); or by applying downward pressure in the abdominal-thoracic area at the end of a regular expiratory phase (chest press). All the foregoing techniques are done with the child in the back-pattern speech posture; all may also be done with the child in the elbow-pattern speech posture, except for the chest press, which is replaced by the back press technique (downward pressure in the lumbar area at the end of an expiratory phase). Except for the chest and back press techniques, all other techniques may also be used in sit- and stand-pattern speech postures.

b. I use four techniques as inspiratory facilitation maneuvers. I call them the arm-lift, leg-roll, accordion, and butterfly techniques. The principle behind the four techniques is similar: respiratory activity enhancement through maximum compression of the thoracic-abdominal area followed by maximum expansion of the area. Because of space limitations, I will describe only the leg-roll and butterfly techniques in some detail. Readers interested in the other breathing therapy techniques should consult appropriate sections of my book on neurospeech therapy.

I do the leg roll with the child lying on a mat or on a massage table. I position myself at the child's feet or side, grasp the child's shins, flex and abduct the legs, press them toward the child's armpits and thereby displace the viscera upward, stretch the diaphragm, and facilitate expiration. Following the expiratory phase, I extend and bring the legs downward to their original position and thereby facilitate inspiration.

The butterfly technique is done with the child sitting on a stool with feet well-placed on the floor and the clinician positioned at the back. I place the child's clasped hands on the back of the child's head, abduct the elbows, fully extend the head and dorsal spine, and thus facilitate inspiration. Following the inspiratory phase, I adduct the child's elbows, flex the head and spine, and bring the head, arms, and shoulders between the child's abducted knees and thus facilitate expiration. I use a rhythm similar to normal vegetative breathing when applying the breathing techniques.

It is through inspiratory reflex and facilitation maneuvers that I hope to improve vegetative breathing in terms of deepening cycles, normalizing bpm's (breaths per minute), and stimulating thoracic participation. The ultimate goal of the breathing techniques is the integration of vegetative breathing into speech breathing.

2. Since it is believed that eating movements contribute to the development of skilled speech movements, I recommend the application of techniques designed to stimulate such movements. I attempt to improve eating movements through the stimulation of the chain of feeding reflexes and the facilitation of actual eating activity.

a. I stimulate the following feeding reflexes: rooting, lip, mouth-opening, tongue, biting, suckle, chewing, and swallow reflexes. I stimulate them when there is a delay in their emergence or when they are weak. (If certain feeding reflexes such as lip, mouth-opening, biting, or suckle have become exaggerated, techniques to facilitate their integration must be employed.) I like to use "natural stimuli" to elicit these reflexes such as a finger, part of a biscuit or cookie, or a pretzel stick. For those readers not familiar with reflex stimulation or integration techniques, I again refer them to the book on neurospeech therapy.

b. For the facilitation of eating movements, I use the following 9-factor approach: nursing, positioning, protecting, priming, transporting, grasping, manipulating, preparing, and swallowing. Space will not allow a detailing of the techniques here, but most of them should be familiar to the reader. Briefly, the nursing factor refers to the recommendation that, whenever possible, nursing should be encouraged as part of any eating therapy program for as long as possible (depending on the condition of the child, different degrees of supplementary feeding may be necessary). The positioning factor refers to establishing proper eating positions (back-pattern, elbow-pattern, and sit-pattern postures) and assisting the child to adjust and orient the body toward the food source (via "therapeutic unbalancing maneuvers"). The protecting factor refers to work to prevent aspiration and choking during eating (e.g., stimulation of various oral protective reflexes such as mouth closure, tongue protrusion, sneeze, cough, palatal and pharyngeal reflexes). The priming factor refers basically to techniques for "muscle priming" or preparing of head control, movements of the jaw, lips, tongue, and swallow before eating. The transporting factor refers to techniques for developing hand-to-mouth, or self-feeding movements (via hand-suckling, hand-holding of bottle, hand-guiding of spoon, and hand-playing with food activities). The grasping factor refers to work on stimulating lip grasping (nipple, cup, straw), tongue grasping (spoon, solid food), and teeth grasping (teeth hold-bite activity). The manipulating factor refers to work on helping the child to adjust the position of the nipple, spoon, morsel, cup, or straw when they are in less than ideal locations in the mouth (via "therapeutic dislocation maneuvers"). The preparing factor refers to techniques for helping the child to draw liquids and semisolids into the mouth and to chew solids already in the mouth (via tongue suckle, lips-suck, upper-lip suckle, and chew preparing maneuvers). Finally, the swallowing factor refers to the stimulation of somatic swallowing (via techniques designed to integrate visceral swallowing).

Regarding eating therapy, I believe that it should be undertaken as soon as possible by the child's family; that as much verbal interaction as possible should take place during the therapy; that the transition from arm and lap feeding to chair feeding and the transition from bottle, to spoon, to cup, to finger feeding should be done as quickly as possible; and that, at each stage of therapy, the child should be provided with only that amount of assistance necessary.

In stimulating the chain of feeding reflexes and eating movements, contributions are made to face-to-face attitudes, speaker-listener movements (rooting reflex), mandibular speech sounds (hand-mouth and mouth-opening reflexes), labial speech sounds (lip reflex), lingua-dental, alveolar, palatal, velar sounds (biting, suckle, chewing, swallow reflexes), and pressure sounds (suckle, swallow, pharyngeal, and palatal reflexes).

Reflexive vocalization includes movement vocalization, hand-to-mouth vocalization, and happy-play vocalization.

1. I elicit movement-associated vocalization, for example, by resisting the child's attempts to raise the head, roll over, or sit up (struggle-movement vocalization) and by creating tasks for the child that require lifting, pushing, pulling, and so on (work-movement vocalization).

2. Since hand-to-mouth vocalization is normally observed in infants and young children during teething, eating, and playing, I recommend that the child's hands be brought together during these activities and that associated vocalization be encouraged.

3. I encourage cooing (vocalization in response to pleasant sensations) and babbling (vocalization for the sake of vocalization) by instructing all those in the child's environment to produce extra amounts of speech when the child is experiencing good feelings, such as when he is being bathed, dried, rubbed, fed, or rocked.

Since the various forms of reflexive vocalization may be viewed as "primary talking," their stimulation should make an important contribution to "true talking."

Skilled Movements

Skilled speech movements emerge from basic speech postures, speech-associated arm-hand movements, and basic speech movements. They represent the integration and elaboration of all subcortical and nuclear mechanisms involved in speech function. It is necessary to stimulate skilled movements directly when there is a delay or retardation in the integration of basic movements. Table 2 summarizes the program of procedures and techniques used for stimulating skilled speech movements.

Listening Movements. Skilled listening movements include se-

Table 2. Summary of Procedures for the Stimulation of Skilled Speech Movements

Procedures	Description
Listening movements	
Selective inhibition of startle	Employ adaptation techniques of overpresentation and gradualism
Localizing	Elicit head localizing through on-effect and stimulating feedback techniques
Perception	Develop speech perception through use of span, discrimination, analysis, synthesis, sequencing, and imagery exercises
Speech movements	
Speech breathing	Use voluntary control exercises and inspiratory facilitation maneuvers
Differentiation	Facilitate through the use of conditioning and isolation maneuvers.
Praxis	Do stimulating-feedback, movement-facilitation maneuvers, and movement exercises
Diadochokinesia	Emphasize speed, duration, and rhythmicity of laryngeal, velar, and articulatory movements

lective inhibition of the startle reflex and facilitation of localizing and speech perception.

Selective inhibition of startle describes the ability of the child to ignore or not to startle to familiar sounds, whereas less familiar and even softer sounds may elicit startle. To help develop selective inhibition capacity, I recommend use of the adaptation techniques of "overpresentation" and gradualism. Overpresentation means the excessive introduction into the child's environment of familiar sounds such as slamming doors, dropping things on the floor, and calling the child's name loudly and unexpectedly. Gradualism means the presentation of the stimuli from progressively decreasing distances, with progressively increasing loudness, and progressing from full warning to no warning.

Localizing describes the ability of the child to orient the head quickly toward the source of speech signals. I do localizing exercises with the child in the back-pattern, elbow-pattern, and sit-pattern speech postures whenever possible. Head localization should be stimulated first to the right and then to the left and first upward and then downward. In choosing stimuli for localizing exercises, I consider the on-effect principle, that is, I select interesting, novel, and changing stimuli. Accordingly, when using voice as the stimulus, I vary pitch, loudness, quality, and time factors. Distances from the stimuli should be progressively increased and loudness levels progressively decreased. When head movements are not spontaneously elicited in the child, I use a therapy partner to initiate and guide these movements until some degree of independent localization on the part of the child is possible (stimulating-feedback technique).

Perception work includes the facilitation of auditory perception in general, but especially of speech signals. I work on span, discrimination, analysis, synthesis, sequencing, and imagery activities. For example, I may work on span by having the child point or eye-localize a progressively increasing number of things named; on discrimination, by having the child signal in some way whether pairs of syllables, words, or phrases are the same or different; on analysis, by having the child identify component syllables of a word or component words of a phrase; on synthesis, by having the child identify words from component syllables (presented with pauses between) or phrases from component words; on sequencing, by having the child unscramble out-of-order syllables of words or words of phrases; and on imagery, by having the child "hear" a response with the "mind's ear" before actually responding.

Speech Movements.   A manifestation of the evolution of skilled speech movements is the emergence of speech breathing, differentiation, praxis, and diadochokinesia.

Speech breathing or "cortical integration" of reflexive breathing is induced through voluntary control exercises and inspiratory facilitation maneuvers.

1.   In voluntary control work, I ask the child to stop or begin breathing upon command, to hold the breath for as long as possible, to deepen breathing, to quicken breathing rate, and to breathe alternately through the nose and mouth.

2.   Inspiratory facilitation maneuvers for speech breathing are based on those described in the section on vegetative breathing, but with air intake and timing modifications. I modify the arm-lift, leg-roll, accordion, and butterfly techniques in the following ways: I lengthen the expiratory phase, and voicing (sustained vowels or syllable strings) is encouraged and stimulated during the procedure, I quicken the inspiratory phase so that its duration is approximately 10 to 15 percent of the entire breathing cycle, and I encourage an oral rather than nasal mode of inspiration.

Differentiation is facilitated through the use of conditioning and isolation maneuvers.

1.   Conditioning is carried out in various speech postures, and includes flexing the upper trunk (front-to-back, side-to-side, rotatory

movement); flexing the head (front-to-back, ear-to-shoulder, rotatory movement); stretching the mandible (extension-flexion movements); stretching, shaking, tapping the lips; spreading and stretching the cheeks away from the dental arch; stretching, shaking, stroking the tongue; and stroking and tapping the velum.

2. I follow conditioning maneuvers with isolation maneuvers. As an example of an isolation maneuver, I will describe mandible isolation from the head: I stand behind the seated child and passively extend and flex the mandible while I provide full hold of the head. Full hold is done by placing the hold-hand across the child's forehead and pressing the head against the clinician's trunk, while the move-hand carries out the mandibular movement. I then ask the child to make the movements spontaneously, with or without assistance, while I maintain the hold. Over time, I provide progressively less hold of the head until the child can voluntarily extend and flex the mandible without associated head movement. Similar maneuvers are used for lip isolation from the head, tongue isolation from the head, and mandible, lip, and tongue isolation from each other. (Details on these maneuvers may be found by referring to appropriate sections of my book on neurospeech therapy.)

Praxis, as used here, is defined as the ability to perform coordinated actions or movements. I call such ability at the level of the larynx, *laryngopraxis,* and at the level of the articulators, *articulopraxis.* To develop effector praxis, I use three techniques: stimulating-feedback, movement-facilitation maneuvers, and movement exercises.

1. Stimulating-feedback maneuvers impose particular sensorimotor speech patterns upon the child's articulatory effector with the expectation that such imposed feedback will facilitate emergence of the respective movements. In other words, I bring the child's articulatory organs through the movements and points of contact associated with the production of key speech sounds for the purpose of generating "therapeutic feedback." Examples: The bilabial pattern of movement and contact is imposed by bringing the child's lips together with the fingers, holding the lips in contact, and asking the child to blow open the contact. The labiodental pattern of movement and contact is imposed by lifting the corners of the child's upper lip with the thumb and index finger of one hand, and exposing the teeth. Then, with the middle three fingers of the other hand placed under the lower lip, and the flat of the thumb placed under the chin for leverage, I raise the lower lip against the upper incisors. I then ask

the child to blow air through the teeth. Labiodental friction sounds may be facilitated by pinching the nostrils. Such a maneuver may first elicit an oral inspiration, which the clinician should allow by releasing the labiodental seal. The seal should be quickly re-established in time for the oral expiration phase through the labiodental contact resulting in labiodental friction. I impose such "labiodental speech breathing" for a number of cycles.

I use similar maneuvers to impose the linguadental pattern of movement and contact (linguadental speech breathing), the lingua-alveolar pattern of movement and contact (lingua-alveolar speech breathing), and the linguavelar pattern of movement and contact (linguavelar speech breathing). I do all the maneuvers with appropriately timed audiovisual sound stimulation, so that the stimulating feedback contains all the important speech-sound sensory dimensions.

2. Movement-facilitation maneuvers are used when there are certain limitations in direction and range of articulatory movements. For this purpose, I use resisted, associated, counter-, reversed, and reflex-movement maneuvers.

a. The resisted-movement maneuver describes neurofacilitation via the application of a challenging force to an intended movement, or what I call the "marshaling effect." Example: I facilitate tongue tip raising and lowering by applying measured resistive pressure with my middle finger against the top of the child's anterior tongue, during efforts to raise the tongue, and with the flat of my thumb against the bottom of the child's anterior tongue during efforts to lower the tongue. I use similar resisted-movement maneuvers to facilitate mandibular flexion-extension and lip rounding-spreading.

b. The associated-movement maneuver describes neurofacilitation via the stimulation of nonintentional smaller movements from intentional larger movements, or what I call the "overflow effect." Example, I facilitate mandibular flexion by having the child begin from a thorax-flexed-forward position and by requesting the child to attempt mouth closure as he extends his trunk into a normal position against measured resistance. I use similar associated-movement maneuvers to facilitate lip rounding-spreading and lingual elevation.

c. The countermovement maneuver describes neurofacilitation via the introduction of a threatening movement requiring an opposing movement, or what I call the "protective effect." Example: I facilitate lip rounding by slowly and steadily spreading the child's lips until a counteracting lip-rounding movement is elicited. I use similar countermovement maneuvers to facilitate mandibular flexion and tongue protrusion.

d. The reversed-movement maneuver describes neurofacilitation via the use of an opposite, facilitatory motion immediately preceding the intended, main motion, or what I call the "coiled spring effect." Example: I facilitate mandibular flexion by having the child attempt to further extend the jaw against measured resistance, and then attempt to close the jaw against measured resistance. I use similar reversed-movement maneuvers to facilitate lip rounding-spreading and tongue elevation.

e. The reflex-movement maneuver describes neurofacilitation via the simultaneous stimulation of a reflex and a voluntary motion that are dependent on the same muscle group, or what I call the "reflex conditioning effect." Example: I facilitate velopharyngeal closure by having the child utter an open vowel, while I simultaneously elicit the palatal reflex.

In order to achieve maximum facilitation of desired movements, I frequently apply movement-facilitation maneuvers in combination.

3. Movement exercises are used to ensure the maximum use of movement potential emerging from stimulating feedback and movement facilitation maneuvers. For this purpose, I employ what I call praxic exercises and sensor-awareness exercises.

a. Praxic exercises involve movements of the larynx, velopharyngeal closure mechanism, and the articulators. Laryngopraxic work describes the serial production of discrete on-off voicing of vowels and diphthongs. I have the child place emphasis on the definition of voice onset and termination movements. An exercise unit is composed of ten cycles of series of ten phonations. Velopraxic work describes the serial production of distinct nasal and non-nasal sounds. I use bilabial /mʌ-bʌ/, lingua-alveolar /nʌ-dʌ/, and linguavelar /ŋ-gʌ/ distinctions. An exercise unit is composed of ten cycles of series of ten bilabial, lingua-alveolar, and linguavelar distinctions. Articulopraxic work involves the production of sets of two-syllable, three-syllable, and four-syllable combinations. I compose sets of syllable combinations including bilabial, labiodental, lingua-alveolar, linguapalatal, and linguavelar sounds. An example of a two-syllable set with the lead syllable /bʌ/ follows: /bʌ-vʌ, bʌ-ðʌ, bʌ-dʌ, bʌ-lʌ, bʌ-dʒ, bʌ-rʌ, bʌ-gʌ/. An exercise unit consists of repeating each pair of the series five times. Other two-syllable sets should be arranged with other syllables serving as lead syllables. As the child progresses, I develop three- and four-syllable sets of exercises.

b. Sensor-awareness exercises are composed of speech forms that are nonspontaneous, reduce rate, and amplify feedback. Among the exercise speech forms are hard-contact speech, exaggerated speech, slow-motion speech, and struggle speech. As examples of struggle speech, I do mandibular-struggle work by having the child speak while the mandible is in a closed position—thus stimulating compensatory movements of the lips and tongue; labial struggle work by having the child speak while the lips remain in an open but immobile state—thus stimulating compensatory movements of the mandible and tongue; and tongue-struggle work by having the child speak while the tongue tip is kept immobile against the upper alveolar ridge—thus stimulating compensatory movements of the mandible and lips.

Diadochokinesia work follows degrees of success with differentiation and praxis tasks. I convert the laryngopraxic, velopraxic, and articulopraxic exercises into laryngodiado, velodiado, and articulodiado exercises by adding the speed component. In addition to the speed or rate of the sets of exercises, I emphasize duration and rhythmicity of performance.

CONCLUDING COMMENTS

I have been concerned with the study and application of developmental neurophysiology to the problem of speech disorders in cerebral palsy for 25 years. During this period, I have seen hundreds of patients, ranging in age from infancy to young adulthood, representing all the major types of cerebral palsy, and showing all degrees of involvement and all levels of motivation. Clearly, the results of my experiences with the approach have warranted my continued use and development of neurospeech theory and therapy over all those years.

Also, all my work with these children has convinced me of the reality of what I call the unmanifested residual potential (URP) factor in neuropathology, that is, the theory that the residual CNS almost always reflects lower than actual potential, and that the way to get at all the child's residual neurophysiology is by challenging it. It is with the goal of reaching each child's maximum URP that I will be developing further the procedures and exercises of neurospeech therapy.

SELECTED REFERENCES

Bobath, K., and Bobath, B. Cerebral Palsy: Part I: Diagnosis and assessment of cerebral palsy; Part II: The neurodevelopmental approach to treatment. In P.

Pearson and C. Williams (Eds.), *Physical Therapy Services in the Developmental Disabilities*. Springfield, Ill.: Charles C Thomas 1972.

Fay, T. The neurophysical aspects of therapy in cerebral palsy. *Archives of Physical Medicine*, 1948, *29:*327–334.

Kabat, H. Central facilitation: The basis of treatment for paralysis. *Permanente Foundation Medical Bulletin*, 1952 *10:*190-204.

Mysak, E. *Neurospeech Therapy for the Cerebral Palsied*. New York: Teachers College Press, Teachers College, Columbia University, 1980.

Stockmeyer, S. An interpretation of the approach of Rood to the treatment of neuromuscular dysfunction. *American Journal of Physical Medicine*, 1967, *46:*900—961.

CHAPTER TWO

TREATMENT OF DEVELOPMENTAL APRAXIA OF SPEECH

Method of Robert W. Blakeley

The suggestions outlined here are to assist with atypical articulation disorders—having multiple errors of phonemic characteristics and often involving vowels—caused by brain damage or cortical dysfunction predating the establishment of voluntary sensorimotor control of the muscles involved in speaking, usually acquired before 3 or 4 years of age. This is a disorder of the voluntary motor system and is not accompanied by a muscle weakness, paralysis, or incoordination, but voluntary oral motor control for nonspeech acts may be affected. I have usually found the disorder to be accompanied by other symptoms and have viewed it as syndrome-like. For example, although it is not a linguistic disorder, language delay may be in evidence. Likewise, it is not a behavioral *anomaly,* but temper tantrums, inflexibility, distractibility, and withdrawal may be present, much of which I believe is due to inability to be understood. Difficulty with verbal sequencing, motorically complex words, and prosody may also be seen. For children under ten years of age, maturation can usually be counted upon as an ally.

THE GENERAL MANAGEMENT PROGRAM

The management of developmental apraxia of speech should be multidimensional and must be directed by the speech-language pathologist. As a profession, we have not heretofore taken full responsibility for this management.

After diagnosis of developmental apraxia of speech, the parents should be advised of the nature and severity of the disorder and given an estimate of the number of years that speech habilitation may take (probably from 3 to 10 years). Even then, as adults, these individuals may continue to have difficulty with motorically complex words. I send reports to the child's physician and teacher if the child is of school age. Communications should relate developmental apraxia of speech to behavioral, language, and academic readiness problems when such factors are relevant. For example, children who are unable to make themselves understood may exhibit aggression, excessive motor activity, or withdrawal. The fact that language comprehension sometimes dramatically exceeds expression may mislead the clinician into assuming that a child has normal intellligence when such may not be the case. Thus, I inform parents that formal intellectual testing to assess academic readiness is advisable prior to their child's enrollment in school.

An Appropriate Mental Set

A significant factor in the management of developmental apraxia of speech is the attitude, or mental set, of the speech-language clinician, and, to no less extent, that of the parents. This factor must be recognized and aired because it relates intimately to the entire habilitative process.

If all children with developmental apraxia of speech were bequeathed to clinicians working in cerebral palsy centers and to the parents of children with cerebral palsy, the management of developmental apraxia of speech would begin with a clinical mental set much closer to the needs of such children. Nevertheless, even such veterans of long-term planning and limited expectation would probably be thrown off balance for a time by these multinormal children with this "idiopathic" speech disorder of such gravity.

Certainly, children having developmental apraxia of speech are generally easier to work with in speech than those with dysarthria of cerebral palsy, and certainly the prognosis for the former is vastly better. The point is that we, as professionals, could cope more ably with developmental apraxia of speech if we adapted quickly, and with less resistance, to the severity and long-term nature of this disorder.

Provide Adequate Speech Intervention Contact

The frequency of professional speech assistance is critical in the habilitation of children with developmental apraxia of speech. This disability calls for all-out attention and deserves serious instruction to the limits of the child's attention and motivation.

When normal children begin their formal education, they do not go to school two or three times a week for just a half-hour at a time, even in kindergarten. Thus, I do not expect to provide speech education for children with developmental apraxia of speech on a cursory basis, for it may be the most important part of their entire education. Daily articulation help is given. If a rigid school schedule interferes with daily contact, then I develop an alternate plan. I may see such children twice daily for 3 days per week, or, intensively, during 8- to 12-week blocks, followed by breaks of a less lengthy block, during which time parents and teachers reinforce the gains made.

The parent and teacher must be used for supportive daily articulation reinforcement activities unless extraordinary problems rule against it.

Clinicians cannot look to, or hope for, remediation by extraordinary technique or scientific breakthrough. The state of the art dictates that they must rely upon the frequency, consistency, and motivation of their instruction for success with developmental apraxia of speech. The extraordinary will be achieved when the clinician provides the appropriate time and motivation for the child.

Prevent Criticism

The number one goal in management of children with developmental apraxia of speech is to foster a satisfactory self-image. Indirect and direct criticism is seen early, when speech intelligibility is lacking or significantly impaired in children. This may start in the home. Parents and relatives must be counseled early about the do's and don'ts of confidence building. For example, there should be no withholding of food or favors because of speech, and no random speech "correction" in the home.

Improve Intelligibility

Much of the apraxic child's management relates directly to improvement in speech intelligibility for its success. Therefore, most of my ongoing energy is expended directly in support of this goal. The child's language (syntax and grammar) does not usually interfere significantly with communication. Impaired intelligibility is more likely to be caused by misarticulation. Thus, any intensive work on syntax and grammar is resisted until it is proved to be of equal or greater interference to intelligibility than are the child's misarticulations.

Reduce Interference of Language with Acceptable Academic Progress

When articulation abnormalities are no longer creating intelligibility problems, and are not evoking significant criticism, then I may address attention to language impairment. If speech intelligibility is not the critical communication problem, I may find it helpful to introduce a language program earlier, particularly when impaired language interferes with acceptable academic progress.

THE INTELLIGIBILITY PROGRAM

There are few hard-and-fast rules for teaching articulation to children having developmental apraxia of speech. There are worthwhile guidelines to consider, but one must be flexible in every instance with every child.

I use the following intelligibility guidelines:

1. Present early-developed consonants.
2. Teach frequently occurring consonants.
3. Introduce visibly produced sounds.
4. Voiceless sounds may be easier than voiced.
5. Use simple whole words or syllables.
6. Use frequently occurring words.
7. Teach a slowed rate as needed.
8. Associate a tactile and visual symbol with sounds.
9. Reinforce movement continuity of sounds (connect syllables) with gestures and intonations.
10. Use knowledge of phonetics to teach sounds and words.
11. Teach vowels early when there is significant interference with intelligibility.

Present early-developed consonants at the outset as these are likely to be easier in all motor aspects, more readily visible, and most likely to be associated with early learned words, e.g., *mama, bye-bye, daddy, no.*

Teach frequently occurring consonants so that a greater intelligibility gap is closed relative to effort expended as the sounds are learned. For example, the three sounds /t/, /d/, /n/ comprise 28.7 percent of all consonant usage (/t/, the most frequently used consonant, occurs 12 percent when compared to all other consonants, whereas /ʒ/ occurs only .06 percent by comparison).

Introduce visibly produced sounds because historically the visual modality in children with developmental apraxia of speech has proved to be helpful. On the other hand auditory stimulation, as a teaching technique, has usually been of limited assistance. Those sounds most visible are /m/, /p/, /b/, /f/, /v/, /θ/, /ð/, /n/, /t/, /d/, /l/, /tʃ/, /dʒ/, /s/, /z/. The least visible consonants are /ɚ/, /r/, /h/, /k/, /g/, /ŋ/.

Voiceless sounds may be easier to teach than those with voice because the latter require additional voluntary motor speech controls. However, I test this in the individual child, so that each is taught according to his or her most rapid learning skills.

Use simple whole words or syllables and then move quickly to phrases and sentences, with much practice up and down this range. The main reason for shifting to syllables from simple words is that prior learning (familiar words) may present strong interference to progress. There need be no strict rule here, except that I avoid lengthy teaching of nonsense syllables without reference to speech meaning. I readily accept single-syllable productions for multisyllable words if these offerings are closer to being correct than habitual productions. However, a strong attempt is made to obtain the correct number of syllables per word.

The teaching of consonants in isolation may be necessary at the outset for some children. Generally, children with developmental apraxia of speech are able to produce most of the isolated sounds correctly. It is the connecting of sounds that is basic to the disorder of developmental apraxia of speech. Nevertheless, productions of some children are so crude that very basic instruction is called for.

Use frequently occuring words so that words learned may more efficiently apply to increased intelligibility. Select words from basic word lists such as the Dolch, and from the child's environment, e.g., words representing food and clothing, the child's first name, names of family members, pets, a close friend, and the teacher's name. Vocabulary that is most meaningful and useful will be carried over first as a general rule. Carrier phrases are helpful to assist in the continuity of adding improved production of vocabulary. For example: I want __; Bobby eats __; I see a __; you tell me __(accompanying this phrase, the child may be required to point to me, to his/her own mouth, and then to the self as gestures to cue use of each word).

Teach a slowed rate of speech to that point where speed is eliminated as an interfering factor to learning articulation. Speed of production may not be a significant problem at the single word level of production, but may become a problem in articulation as phrases and sentences are attempted. The prolongation of vowels is one helpful means to slow the rate. The slowing of rate for successful production of phoneme clusters, as in "truck," may be achieved by adding the /ə/, hence /tərʌk/. The effect is to allow time for motoric control of two consonants occurring side by side.

Associate a tactile and visual symbol with sounds to reinforce their presence. For example, I may squeeze the child's lips together to provide a tactile cue for /p/ or /b/. The plosiveness may be symbolized then by rapidly opening my fingers and pulling my hand away (in association with my production), or by expelling air against the back of the child's hand. After some initial success with this technique, the same set of tactile and visual gestures carried out by me on my own body will act as cues for the child to remember the phonetic gestures.

The sharp end of a broken Q-tip rubbed against the tongue tip and maxillary alveolar ridge will reinforce the articulatory contact for /t/, /d/, /n/. Similarly, an index finger pressed firmly against the child's upper lip, under the nose, during production (by me and the child) of these same sounds will reinforce the articulatory place of contact and thus will assist with movement. Pressure applied well under the child's chin, upward and toward the base of the tongue, will reinforce back-of-tongue (/k/, /g/, /ŋ/) productions in a like manner. The child soon learns to make the reinforcing gesture independently, or when cued.

It is helpful to articulate syllables in chorus with the child. Later, I mouth sounds, as the child moves toward such sounds, to provide a strong articulatory cue. In most of these examples the child uses visual imitation along with auditory and tactile cues. Written symbols can also serve as reminders for articulatory gestures, and a child may even learn to "talk along" the chalk board as a parallel walk takes him/her by a series of sound symbols, e.g., /aɪ – wɔk – baɪ/. In such instances the symbols for vowel sounds should be those which the child will be (or has been) taught in school, so that confusion related to reading may be avoided.

When a child can read, the use of written material is a helpful visual stimulus. Problem sounds, syllables, or words may be underlined or encircled. The child may also be taught to time gestural or tactile cues with the production of these visual cued sounds or words.

Reinforce movement continuity of sounds (connect syllables) with gestures and intonation in ways similar to the previous guideline for using tactile and visual symbols. However, in the present guideline, syllables are cued by association with movement and tone shift.

Gross body gesture, such as swinging of the arm or tapping the table, is timed to provoke inclusion or connecting of syllables. The gesture serves as the reminder for sound movement (sequencing).

In a similar manner, the use of contrasting tones, or tone changes, as a timing technique, or reminder, is helpful to some children. This technique may be combined with others, such as gross body gestures. For example, in teaching the diphthong /aɪ/, a vowel sequence, for the personal pronoun, *I*, one may start with a normal voice for /ɑ/ and glide, in almost an octave shift, upward to /ɪ/ (only I would substitute the vowel /i/ strongly here, as it provides greater contrast to /ɑ/ than does /ɪ/). A rising hand gesture could be used at this point, thus doubling the cue value.

Use knowledge of phonetics to teach syllables and words because children with developmental apraxia of speech usually produce phonemes in a rudimentary fashion. Two of three, or all three, phonetic characteristics (place of production, acoustic characteristic, and voicing factor) may be missing, or in error.

If sounds are nasalized inappropriately and difficult to alter, I manually occlude the child's nose to force the sound out of the mouth. If nasalization with nasal emission persists as part of the apraxia, then I use a temporary obturator (speech prosthesis) to control this aspect of misarticulation. It can be removed when orality has been learned.

All plosives, and many other sounds, may be taught and experienced in syllable chains by manipulating the child's tongue or lips during phonation, or during voiceless exhalation of air. This can be done with the fingers or with a tongue stick as follows:

/m/, /b/—Manually open and close the child's lips during humming or voicing orally.

/p/—Manually open and close the child's lips during blowing. Ask the child to add and delete voice to obtain syllables (model this for the child).

/n/, /d/, /l/—Lift the child's tongue tip alternately with a tongue stick while the child is humming or voicing orally. If the child can start /n/ with the tongue tip up, but cannot lower it, do this for the child.

/t/—Lift the child's tongue tip alternately with a tongue stick while the child is extending /h/. Ask the child to add and delete voice to obtain syllables.

/t/, /d/, /n/, /l/—May also be taught by manually elevating the tongue tip to the bottom of the upper lip. This provides a new or different tactile sensation and each sound is made more visible. The tongue tip can be brought back into the mouth in stages later on.

/k/, /g/, /ŋ/—During exhalation of air (such as during production of /h/), or during oral phonation, I push the tongue posteriorly with a tongue stick until the dorsum makes contact with the soft palate, then I lower the tongue immediately (withdraw the stick slightly) for /k/ or /g/. I retain the tongue in the elevated position, to force the sound into the nose, for /ŋ/.

/j/—Introduce with the vowel /i/ and move to another vowel according to the word desired, e.g., /i→u/ = /ju/; /i → æ/ = /j æ/, etc.

/w/—Introduce with the vowel /u/ and move to another vowel according to the word desired, e.g., /uʌt/ = /wʌt/; /uʌn/ = /wʌn/, etc.

/s/, /ʃ/, /tʃ/—Ask the child to "suck air" out of the end of a fountain straw "with the end of your tongue" (hold the straw one-half inch or so from the teeth). I model for the child. When the acoustic effect of a sibilant is produced anteriorly in the mouth, I ask the child to make the air "come back out and go through the straw," then, to go "back and forth" through the straw. Eventually this sibilant (/s/) can be shaped by occluding the teeth and forcing the lips back into a smile, or by rounding the lips manually (/ʃ/) and pushing the tongue tip posteriorly with a Q-Tip. The affricate (/tʃ/) may be aided by elevating the tongue tip with a tongue stick. A vowel should be added as soon as any success is achieved. I do not identify most of the sounds noted in this section until they have been successfully produced.

Teach vowels early when there is significant interference with intelligibility; otherwise I delay this activity in favor of more serious needs in the hope that maturation will provide some advantage. Combinations of two vowels, diphthongs, usually provide the most difficulty because each of these constitutes a movement sequence.

I am alert to the fact that attempted production of certain vowels or diphthongs may cause adjacent consonant errors. This may mislead me into focusing on the consonant as the problem.

To assist in the teaching of vowels I observe my own mouth in a mirror during production. Thereafter, I manually place the child's tongue and lips into like posture and position, then ask the child to "make a noise" (providing the correct auditory stimulus may cause immediate shifting of oral postures and, thus, the habitually incorrect auditory response). Even during neutral phonation, the child's tongue and lips can be manipulated into different vowels.

CONFERENCE AND REVIEW

The need for periodic conferences with the parents and teachers of children with developmental apraxia of speech cannot be overstated.

Their frequent frustration with the child's slow progress may lead to behaviors that threaten to undermine the overall program or some of its goals. Again, the clinician must serve in the authority role regarding the disorder, as the manager of the speech and language program, and as the motivator of the child, the parents, and the teacher.

SELECTED REFERENCES

Blakeley, R. *Screening Test for Developmental Apraxia of Speech*. Tigard, Oregon: C.C. Publications, Inc., 1980.

Rosenbek, J., and Wertz, R. A review of 50 cases of developmental apraxia of speech. *Language, Speech and Hearing Services in Schools*, 1972, 3:23-33.

Rosenbek, J., Hanson, R., Baughman, C., and Lemme, M. Treatment of developmental apraxia of speech: A case study. *Language, Speech and Hearing Services in Schools*, 1974, 5:13-22.

Yoss, K., and Darley, F. Developmental apraxia of speech in children with defective articulation. *Journal of Speech and Hearing Research*, 1974, 17:399-416.

Yoss, K., and Darley, F. Therapy in developmental apraxia of speech. *Language, Speech and Hearing Services in Schools*, 1974, 5:23-31.

CHAPTER THREE

COMMUNICATION SYSTEMS FOR THE CHILD WITHOUT SPEECH

Method of Judy K. Montgomery

Children may fail to develop oral speech for three reasons: severe developmental and cognitive disabilities, severe neurological impairments such as cerebral palsy, or a combination of these. Further, children may *lose* the ability to speak, owing to traumatic head injury or similar cerebral insult. The techniques described here are primarily for training a congenitally nonoral child to use an augmentative-communication system. The same steps could be followed for an acquired condition in a child, with some adjustments made for the rehabilitative advantage of his/her normal acquisition of speech and language. Since there are numerous types of communication systems available to the nonoral child, the strategies outlined here will be common to all of them. I have found that there are more similarities than differences in the training models used for these systems. The most significant difference is the preprogrammed vocabulary versus the custom vocabulary. Again, I have found it to be most beneficial to use a modification of this approach to teach any vocabulary or system.

COMPARISON WITH AN AUGMENTATIVE-COMMUNICATION SYSTEM FOR ADULTS

There is a significant difference between the strategies for teaching a nonoral child and a nonoral adult. Although major portions of the two strategies coincide, the sequence, timing, and content are vastly different. The reason for this divergence is critical to the development of communication. The nonoral child, unlike the adult or individual with late onset of the condition, needs an augmentative system for two reasons: (1) to interact with others, and (2) to learn language.

Without an oral feedback system, the young child fails to go through the normal language-acquisition process. Lacking speech, he/she is unable to question, respond, rehearse, rephrase, refuse, release frustrations, etc. This greatly affects the language-learning process. If the dysarthria is compounded by cognitive limitations, the cycle is further upset. Therefore, the augmentative-communication system must function as both an interaction tool and a language-learning vehicle.

SELECTION BASED ON FIVE FACTORS

The selection of an appropriate nonoral system is based on a child's skills in five areas: motor skills, cognition, visual and auditory perception, psycholinguistic abilities, and communication needs. The assessment of these factors is described in detail in several available books (Yoder and Reichle, 1977; Montgomery, 1980). I do a task analysis of the skills needed for a particular system being considered. If the child exhibits at *least* 50 percent of these skills at the assessment time, I proceed with the training. If less than 50 percent are observed, either the child is intensively coached in specific skills needed, or an entirely different system is considered through the same task analysis method.

THE ROLE OF AN INTERDISCIPLINARY TEAM

Although the primary responsibility for the treatment of a communication disorder lies with the speech-language pathologist, an augmentative system often extends the professionals' boundaries. That is, motor skills, cognitive and academic levels, and perceptual areas are equally important to successful use of the system. I utilize the expertise of many others when teaching or developing a new system. I ask the occupational or physical therapist to assist with positioning, perception, and gross and fine motoric abilities. I rely on the special education teacher to develop academic goals, select reading approaches, and integrate the child's system into a classroom repertoire. The parent or care provider is vital to the motivation, personalization, and carryover aspects of the process. From time to time, I call on medical and psychological personnel, or social workers.

Since the child learns language by interacting with a variety of people, I find it necessary to manipulate the environment as well. Facilitating peer interactions, cluing significant others into the child's response mode, and generally creating communication events when none might naturally occur—all speed up the acquisition.

ESTABLISHING PRELINGUISTIC SKILLS

When I work with the very young nonoral child or the severely developmentally delayed individual, I work toward three goals: (1) developing communicative intent, (2) establishing a means to indicate, and (3) offering an environment for interaction.

I guide the nonresponding child into a series of environmental confrontations that shape his responses. Looking, listening, and reaching activities promote the basic forms of choice making. Handing toys back and forth, following my line of visual regard, searching for a hidden object are all precursor activities to communication as we know it. I utilize the stages of motor patterns according to Piaget to facilitate the next higher level of physical response. I believe, along with others in the field, that communication systems cannot be expected to be effective as interaction tools until the child reaches Piagetian stage 6 (18 to 24 months: naming, substituting, recognizing two-dimensional symbols).

I observe and facilitate the following pre-linguistic actions in the young child:

1. Mutual attending and eye contact
2. Showing off objects
3. Pointing to objects
4. Using objects to act on objects
5. Using objects to attract another's attention
6. Turn-taking

Next, I plan therapy around the age-typical motor and language patterns of the young child under two years of age. He uses language to get his needs met, comment upon the here and now, and imitate those around him. By encouraging these activities, I utilize the other team members to respond meaningfully to the nonoral child. Expecting near-age-level mental reactions from severely dysarthric children helps to mitigate the effects of years without speech.

I try to develop the concepts of *yes/no* or *want/don't want* throughout this period. I recognize that the words *yes* and *no* carry much less meaning for the young child than *want/don't want*. Again, developmentally, *no* enters the receptive and expressive vocabulary of the intact child long before *yes*. *No* is a word he hears often and needs to say to impact his environment. Vocally, it occurs by 16 to 20 months of age. When teaching the nonoral system, I anticipate a motor-defined *no!* response long before a *yes*. I do not, therefore, introduce it as a dichotomy. The use of *No!* in whatever form the augmentative system allows, is an important benchmark. *Yes,* or the affirmative, will emerge later.

Toys are a great source of stimulus for this stage. I use commercially available and custom-made toys, as well as modifications for severely motor-handicapped children. These help to develop object permanence, cause and effect, sequence, anticipation, turn-taking, logical thinking, etc. The language associated with the play is an excellent model for the child; the reinforcement is immediate and the activity shadows typical, interactive, prelinguistic play.

INTRODUCING A RESPONSE MODE

At this point, I have completed the pretesting, assessed or facilitated the prelinguistic skills, and selected the appropriate system. The next step is to teach the response mode needed to operate the system. For example, if the child will use a communication board, the response mode will be finger-pointing, If he used an electronic visual display, it may be scanning. If he uses a microcomputer, it is depressing keys. If he uses a voice synthesizer, he may need to activate touch-sensitive 1-inch squares with a pointer. Whatever motor skill is required—whether appropriate visual tracking or sustained pressure or repeated movements—must be taught.

Children appear to learn much of the operation of a communication device by actual experience, not demonstration. Talking through the process is much less effective than doing it. I often take the unit or system home with me several times to learn the operation, so that I can teach it without having directions in front of me or without being surprised by a quirk for which I am not prepared. It is not uncommon for a child to seemingly "play" with an electronic device for awhile before he uses it more seriously. Most of us learn faster and more thoroughly with a trial-and-error method than with instructions. I like to allow the child some unstructured time with the more complex types of augmentative aids. An aide, paraprofessional, or care provider can sit with a child and monitor the early experimentation. This playfulness is a positive sign of the child's interest in manipulation. He must eventually learn to manipulate language to get what he wants, and this serves as early practice.

Sometimes a child is passive, fails to respond at all, or is unable to choose, It may be necessary to teach choice-making in a step-by-step manner before any progress can be made. The following sequence has been effective in moving a child from this point to a two-dimensional picture/symbol language board:

1. Always work within a training frame to teach organization and control the stimuli.

2. Start with concrete three-dimensional objects. Place one to three items in front of the child, Ask him to "show me cup" or "get the comb." Give him the object if he correctly locates it. It is important for him to actually manipulate it at this stage. Keep changing objects and adding to the ones shown. Gradually add up to ten choices.

3. At the next stage, the child is asked to "find the *ball*" or "get *the hamburger*." This time when he locates it, he is rewarded with an identical object from out of sight. Advance to ten choices.

4. Next, the child selects a named object (e.g., "show me the toothbrush") by pointing to the accompanying photograph of it. He gets to manipulate the correct item taken from the out-of-sight area. Advance to ten choices.

5. Next, he gets the object only when he finds the picture of the stated object. All of the three-dimensional clues are taken away. This transition can be very slow. When it is accomplished, the child has entered the symbolic or representational stage.

6. Next, the picture/photos are reduced to fit on one board. Selection should now be self-reinforcing and require the actual object on an intermittent basis. Rewards can become more socially oriented, instead of physical.

The items selected for this training, or any portion of the augmentative system, must have significance in the child's life. I have seen many systems that are designed for the *adult,* not the child. Boards that are all pictures of daily physical needs—eating, sleeping, toileting—are of little interest to children. The activities will occur whether they choose them or not. Social or personal experiences are highly motivating. Pictures or symbols of favorite toys, unusual animals, special foods, or novel experiences (a water balloon that burst in therapy once became a real motivation!) can make the difference. The greater the involvement, the stronger the child's learning and desire to participate.

All activities should be introduced from left to right to reinforce visual scanning and eventual reading. Again, the very young or delayed child may need to have all activities presented in the plane parallel with his body. The upright presentation precedes the table-top presentation, developmentally. Gradually, the board or pictures can be tipped at various angles and finally lie flat on the table. Two-by four-inch boards with a slit down the middle function as a picture or card holders. These allow the student to view stimuli at a 10 to 15 percent slant from the vertical.

Selecting the appropriate vocabulary for a communication system requires some thought and experimentation. It is not unusual to change the words or symbols or entire approach several times. There is no right way, only a series of reasonable choices for the clinician to make. For the nonreader there are:

Objects
Photographs
Pictures (color)
Pictures (black and white)
Line drawings
Rebus symbols
Blissymbols
Non-slip
Personal symbols
Any combination of the above

For the reader there are:

Traditional orthography (alphabet)
Punctuation
Phonetic symbols
Syllables
Numbers
Number codes
Any combination of these

The clinician will introduce the vocabulary system felt to be the most beneficial to the child for learning the communication system. The vocabulary may be changed when the system is learned and greater complexity is desired. If a reading student uses a clinician-made language board, for instance, the units of information must be functional for conversation and academics.

It is at this juncture that I divide my strategy into preprogrammed and custom vocabulary. If the system selected for the child has a built-in or preprogrammed vocabulary, I begin to teach it in small increments, according to his environmental needs and the normal acquisition of word forms. If the system requires that I design a vocabulary, I add words or symbols gradually, also dependent upon environment and normal order. Now, it is possible to combine all the elements that have been taught into one pattern—the physical response mode, the choice-making, the vocabulary, and the intent. I expect a plateau for many children at this point. Some can move swiftly to the next learning, but others require considerable practice to turn this into a viable system. If repeated sessions at this point (more than 3 months) reveal little or no change, I review the obstacle and consider modification or reintroduction to another system. Children are growing and changing at a rate that can outdistance or circumvent our best attempts to meet their needs. Physical changes, in particular, may cause you to change approaches. Cognitive limits will be very obvious at this point, if a child fails to combine and use the learnings. I also rely on the other team members, at this stage, to evaluate an especially long plateau.

DEVELOPMENT OF SENTENCE STRUCTURE

Next, I plunge into word or symbol stringing resulting in kernel sentences and simple language structures. Children without speech have not orally produced a string of words followed by longer and longer utterances. They have not ordered and reordered words to get the exact meaning intended. They have not stored information to call up in new situations, or made up words just for the fun of saying them, or gotten excited reactions from parents when something cute or surprising was said. Without these experiences, we do not know whether they can internally construct sentences they will never utter. We do not know whether they use a telegraphic style, mentally as well as physically, when they are hampered by severe dysarthria. Experience has shown that syntactical structures can be most effectively taught to these children, using the developmental sequence of neurologically intact children.

Briefly, I introduce the vocabulary with nouns followed by locatives, action verbs, and possessive pronouns. As the sentences are lengthened, I add adverbs, adjectives, and a few propositions. Intransitive verbs (is, are) are taught as helpers to the word they precede (Tom *is* sick). Negation is taught first as the word preceded by no ("no Mommy," "no car") for meaning and then transferred to the correct form ("Mommy went home," "the car is gone."). Pronouns other than *I* are of questionable use to the nonoral person, since they must immediately identify the proper noun to the receiver anyway. This compounds the interchange and increases the time for what could have been a short meaningful exchange. For example:

Child on language board: She told me to keep it until tomorrow.
Receiver: "Keep what?"

Child on board: The library book.
Receiver: "Who told you?"
Child on board: His mother.
Receiver: "Whose mother said that?"
Child on board: Jimmy's.
Receiver: "Oh. Now I see what you mean!" etc.

For this reason, pronouns are carefully taught as words referring to proper nouns in the same written paragraph. They are more useful in written communications than in face-to-face ones, where time is of the essence. When using pictures or symbols, I include a place on a language board for a thought, word, or idea that has not been depicted. This allows the child to signal that he has a *new* thought, or at least a need or interest, that I overlooked in organizing the board. Although I have to guess the word from the child's clues, it proceeds faster than without the special frame.

Strategies for language use are taught next. Systems within a system are necessary to signal ideas more quickly—*opposite of, similar to, start over, I'm spelling now,* etc. These are organized on the board.

I try to use the communication system conversationally every time we have a session. This establishes the system as more than a work tool for the child, and increases my understanding of his abilities and interests. I try to encourage the flow of conversation—*I talk, you talk*—to instill the give-and-take nature of communication. Nonoral children have been talked *at* for so long that they need many opportunities to participate and influence others with language. I let them see the *power* of communcation, that things can and do happen *because* they communicate. This cannot be overemphasized for the severely handicapped child who has so little independence.

When teaching communication-system users, I remember that structure is secondary to function. When initiating or responding, their meaning is more important than their grammar. I react first to the message, and only secondarily to the structures. Language modeling or language expansion methods can be effective ways to teach the corrected syntax *after* the meaning is appreciated.

Finally, I use language development materials commercially prepared for the new response system of the nonoral child. I determine what skill I need to remediate, then locate available resources, and adjust them as needed. Since a normal developmental sequence is utilized in this approach, the modifications are usually in the response mode, timing, and interest level. Ideas are listed in *A Training Guide For the Child Without Speech,* California State Department of Education, 1980.

CHARTING THE FUNCTIONS OF LANGUAGE

I have found that we can become preoccupied with the "getting information" aspect of communication. Children, in particular, use their language for many purposes, and will turn off if a communication system appears to be only a way for the clinican to get information. I attempt to survey the child's use of his existing language and looks for ways to expand it. It is helpful to refer to the Yoder/Reichle list of universal functions of language and select additional goals for the nonoral communicator. It is just as crucial to have entertainment options for a communication system as information options. The functions of language in the communication process, according to Yoder and Reichle, are:

1. Giving information
2. Getting information
3. Describing events
4. Getting listeners to:
   • do something
   • believe something
   • feel something
5. Expressing one's own:
   • intentions
   • beliefs
   • feelings
6. Indicating desire for further communication
7. Entertainment
8. Learning new behavior:
   • rehearsal
   • reinforcement
   • feedback
9. Interactional
10. Personal gratification

CLASSROOM AND HOME CARRYOVER

I work closely with the special educator and parent to ensure the continuity of the new communication system. Strong habits of parent and child must often be altered to move away from immature responses into more complex and demanding language structures. These must be payoffs for the child in the form of increased attention and social rewards. The peers must be an integral part of the classroom scene, so that the nonoral communicator does not feel singled out for excessive work. Children are highly manipulative, and system users must be given the same opportunities to succeed or fail in their attempts to deal with each other.

I know that many family and classroom routines can be restructured to allow the child to use his augmentative system. I keep a list of the environmentals in which he is most successful, and why. I gradually add new people, places, and items to his experiences as an aid user. At times, this requires spending additional time with the parents—teaching them how to operate the system, trouble shoot it if necessary, and expand their child's language base. Transferring the skills to academics is usually a joint effort with the special educator and/or psychologist.

MEASURING EFFECTIVENESS

I measure effectiveness in three ways—objectively, with tests; subjectively, with interviews; and personally, with observations. I find that communication skills seem to become a gradual combination of a formal augmentative system and an informal gesture, oral, mime system. The individual develops a style of communication use that is uniquely his own—just as we do with speech. Measuring the effectiveness of this challenges me to gauge the relative improvement of overall communication that can be attributed to the system. I test in all the cognitive, psychomotor, and perception areas tapped before. I measure the size and range and use of the vocabulary. I compute the speed, duration, and number of occurrences of the new system use. I question and survey others to determine their ideas on how, when, and where the child interacts. Finally, I interview the child himself, if possible, to ask him what he thinks of the system and what changes he would like to see made.

These facts are gathered and reviewed to decide what alterations or extensions need to be made. Sometimes an additional system with another output mode is necessary, when, for example, a child needs to have hard copy output for test-taking in the classroom. When adolescents want to use the telephone, similar modifications must be made.

Finally, overall intelligibility is rated by a group of three persons who do not typically interact with the system user. The child "reads" 10 prepared utterances that the raters write down, independently. Each utterance is repeated twice. Oral speech can be used to enhance whatever system is operating. The raters' responses are tallied for accuracy, and the resulting number divided by total utterances is the percentage of intelligibility. This measure may not be possible for very young or significantly delayed children.

SELECTED REFERENCES

Montgomery, J. *Non-Oral Communication: A Training Guide for the Child Without Speech*. Sacramento, CA.: State Department of Education, 1980.

Oakander, S. *Language Board Instruction Kit*. 1980 (Printed by and available from the Non Oral Communication Center, 9675 Warner Avenue, Fountain Valley, CA. 92708).

Vanderheiden, G., and Grilley, K. (Eds.). *Non-Vocal Communication Techniques and Aids for the Severely Physically Handicapped*. Baltimore: University Park Press, 1976.

Yoder, D.E., and Reichle, J.E. In P. Mittler (Ed.), *Research to Practice in Mental Retardation*. Vol. 2, 1977.

PART TWO:
APRAXIA AND DYSARTHRIA IN ADULTS

CHAPTER FOUR

TREATMENT FOR APRAXIA OF SPEECH IN ADULTS

Method of John C. Rosenbek

Treatment for the apraxic talker is like a stream. It surges, gurgles, eddies, and, at times, seems ready to dry up altogether. To describe that treatment in a chapter is no more possible than is capturing a stream in a bottle. Nonetheless, a chapter can give a sense of that treatment just as the bottled water might give an idea of the stream's temperature, color, and occupants. This is our bottle. It will have nothing of real treatment's motion and force. It is intended only as a sample, and to provide some notion about what it might be that brushes against one's legs as he stands in the stream.

GETTING SPEECH STARTED

Apraxic talkers have a *good* prognosis for recovery of functional communiction *without* treatment and they have an *excellent* prognosis with it. With the severely apraxic speaker—most begin that way and some remain so for months or years—the clinician will want to get some speech started in the first few sessions. Initially, we use a prosaic set of stimuli and methods. If they work, we exult and then press on. If they fail, we re-examine our diagnosis, because even chronic apraxic talkers can learn, although for some the learning stops after only a few sessions. This chapter is not for those who cannot learn to talk at all (these patients are probably globally aphasic), or who master only a few sounds or syllables. Such patients deserve an alternative mode of communication, and, failing that, they deserve freedom from all treatment. The material in this chapter is for those with sufficient physiological support for speech to enable them to once again learn to speak some, or all, of what is on their minds.

The Stimuli

Our first stimuli, whether the patient's condition is acute or chronic, are not /a/, /pʌpʌpʌ/, or "gingerbread." Rather, they are **49** explanations of who we are, why we have been summoned, and what we can offer. Only when the patient says he is willing do we have him join in some testing that helps us to help him.

Testing begins with meaningful stimuli, not only because patients seem to appreciate it, but because apraxic motor systems respond better to meaning than to nonsense. We ask them to count. We have them try to imitate common CV and CVC words, and more familiar words, like their names and home towns. And despite the litany on apraxia of speech, which says that apraxic talkers make more errors as stimuli increase in length, we have even severe patients try to imitate a few simple sentences such as "I love you." Patients some-times refuse to obey group trends, and we have evaluated more than one who could say some long sentences better than some shorter ones, and who could say words better than individual sounds. And, regardless of whether the patient has said anything up to this point, we end the first session by determining the stimulability of the vowels, beginning with /i/, /u/, and /a/, and the consonants, beginning usually with the plosives /p/, /t/, and /k/. Where one begins such stimulability testing, however, is less important than that, once begun, it is sys-tematic and thorough. Stimulability testing indicates which sounds the patient is likely to relearn quickly, and in what environments.

As a result of such testing the clinician usually has a variety of vowels, consonants, syllables, and words that can be used as the raw materials for building functional communication. Using methods to be described, we try to stabilize these stimuli and combine them into longer, functional units. Some patients, however, are barely stimulable, and it is obvious that—at least at first—each sound and syllable is going to be learned only after sweaty, protracted labor. Under such conditions we choose to concentrate first on frequently occurring sounds in initial position because these sounds can improve communication, even if they are never learned in other positions, and even if less frequently occurring sounds never appear.

The Methods

Imitation is parsimonious, and we begin with it. The instruction is merely to "watch me, listen to me, and do what I do." If a response does not appear within three to five repetitions, we add *phonetic placement*. Phonetic placement comprises a host of traditional ap-proaches, including description of what is to be done; graphs, pictures, or other representations of what is to be done; and manipulation of the articulators. We seldom use graphs or pictures, but we make liberal use of both description and manipulation. We describe how the lips, jaw, and tongue should be shaped and positioned, and we try to create verbal associations for the sounds. For example, /p/ is like a bubble (as most phoneticians would agree), /s/ sounds like the high-pitched sound of air escaping from a tire, and /ʃ/ is what one is supposed to be in a hospital zone.

Manipulation of the patient's articulators may be just the addition to imitation that gets the severe patient to make a sound he has otherwise been unable to make. Analyzing what the patient does as he tries to make particular sounds, and comparing those attempts to what normals do, will give the clinician clues about what to manipulate. To get an /a/ for example, he may merely have to depress the patient's jaw. At other times, he may have to mold the entire sound. A /k/ may require him to position the jaw, mold the lips, inhibit the tongue tip, and facilitate the tongue back. These manipulations take an octopus' agility, if not the same number of appendages, but are usually worth it. Once a sound returns, the manipulations can be faded.

Sounds that fail to return, regardless of how hard the clinician works, can be ignored during treatment's early days in the hope (usually one that is subsequently realized) that they will appear spontaneously, or will be easier to treat later on. If a troublesome sound is crucial because of its frequency or for some other reason, however, the clinician—instead of relying on hope—can try *derivation*. In this method, something the patient can do is modified to yield something he cannot. The derivation materials may be either speech or nonspeech movements. As examples, a sound such as /u/ can be modified to yield a /k/, an /s/ can be made to yield /ʃ/ by adding lip rounding, a /t/ may be modified to produce an /s/, and nonverbal movements such as biting, blowing, and sucking can be modified to yield a variety of stop plosives and fricatives. Other examples are as numerous as clinicians.

KEEPING SPEECH GOING

As sounds begin to emerge, we do three things more or less simultaneously. We combine shorter units into longer ones—sounds into syllables and words, and words into sentences. We introduce delays between something we do and something the patient does. We have him practice progressively more competitive stimuli. We do not measure our delay intervals with a stop watch, but we do force the patient to delay his imitations of our model for progressively longer periods. And as his control improves, we ask him not only to delay, but to respond two or several times consecutively without further help from us. During the delays, we ask him to mull the target over in his mind and plan how he will say it, and during each production, we ask the patient to focus on the sound and feel of correctness. If a response disintegrates, we return to simple imitation, only to reintroduce delays and consecutive responses when the response is once again intact.

Competition among stimuli is created by *contrasts*. Instead of having a patient practice a single target or sound, we have him move back and forth between one or more pairs of sounds, each pair being a contrast. A contrast may involve a vowel and consonant, two vowels, two consonants, or a singleton consonant and a consonant cluster. Specific contrasts for each patient can be derived from an evaluation of his errors and abilities, and from phonetic principles about the relative similarity of pairs of sounds. Some, such as /m/ and /a/, are relatively easy because the two sounds have few common features; others, such as between the voiced and voiceless members of a cognate pair, are more difficult. Perhaps the most difficult of all is between a target and the sound the patient substitutes for that target. For example, difficult pairs of stimuli for a patient who substitutes /t/ for /k/ in word-final position would be "bait-bake," "bite-bike," and "beet-beak." Manner, place, voicing, and oral-nasal distinctions can all be re-established by the enlightened use of contrasts.

INCREASING INDEPENDENCE

Once the apraxic talker has begun to recall how sounds are made, to contrast those sounds with others, and to combine them into words and short phrases, traditional methods like imitation, placement, and derivation can be replaced by methods that slow connected speech and heighten rhythm and stress profiles. The two methods we use most frequently for these purposes are gestural reorganization and the contrastive stress drill.

Gestural Reorganization

Luria (1970) described a set of techniques for treating the sequelae of nervous system damage, which he called *intersystemic reorganization*. In his view, intersystemic reorganization resulted when something unique was introduced into the performance of damaged behavior. As an example, he described modifying a parkinsonian patient's festinating gait by having him step on each of a set of parallel black lines as he walked. Luria's idea spurred us to begin introducing unique stimuli and behaviors into the act of speaking to measure their palliative effect on apraxic speech. The addition that seems most promising is simple, rhythmic gesturing. We have dubbed our program, which teaches the patient to combine speaking and gesturing, *gestural reorganization*. The method is roughly divisible into three steps, but only the first two are necessary.

Selecting and Practicing the Gestures. In the first step, clinician and patient choose a gesture such as tapping against the table top, lap board, or arm of a wheel chair. The two requirements for such a gesture are that it be simple and within the patient's ability, either with or without practice. Whether the gesture should be performed with the arm, foot, or body; with the left or right side; and whether the patient should learn a single, stereotyped gesture or a variety of different ones, can be decided after diagnostic teaching. In our view it is appropriate—even mandatory—to have the patient practice whatever gesture is ultimately selected, so that he can vary its stress and rhythm at will. It accomplishes nothing, except further degradation of speech, to have the patient combine something he can barely do— gesture—with something he cannot do—talk. This first step, then, must be stood upon long enough so that the patient learns to control his gesturing. When he can, we move to step two.

Combining Gesture and Speech. The gesture(s), once learned, can be paired systematically with speaking. No rules govern the exact pairing. Usually, we find it best to begin by providing a model; therefore we tap and talk while the patient watches and listens. If he needs it, we next take his hand in ours and guide him through the tapping, while urging him to speak simultaneously with us. As he can, we allow him to tap and/or talk independently, intervening only if one or the other falters. At first, we usually have the patient accompany each syllable with a tap. As he improves, we may begin fading the tap so that it occurs only on key words.

The greatest danger is moving too quickly. The patient's tendency is to use as few gestures as possible; the clinician's is to allow it. Neither is appropriate. Even if gestures do nothing as grand as reorganizing neuromotor control, they do slow a patient down, heighten rhythm and stress profiles, and they can serve to remind the patient that he must attend to each syllable of an utterance. To allow sloppy, inconsistent gesturing is to defeat the program, and perhaps the patient. Once the gesture and speech duet has been learned, the patient can profit from as many repetitions of as many different stimuli as time allows.

Fading the Gesture.   This step is optional. Hearing aids, canes, and glasses are accepted treatments for chronic disability; gestures can be, too. On the other hand, the gesture can be faded if speech is adequate without it. Usually the clinician need do nothing spectacular. Patients march (and gesture) to their own drummers, and most will begin abandoning gestures as they feel they can. This fading, if it is appropriate, can be hastened by the clinician's having the patient alternately gesture and not gesture, all the while trying to preserve equal speech adequacy in both conditions. Many patients arrive at a sane compromise. They gesture only when the message is especially important, or when they get in trouble.

The Contrastive Stress Drill

A contrastive-stress drill (Fairbanks, 1960) is nothing more than a question-and-answer dialogue. The rationale for its use is that primary stress, and the rhythmic accompaniment of that stress, seem to facilitate apraxic speech movements. Apraxic talkers, for example, are better able to articulate primarily stressed words than those with lesser forms of stress. Whether it is the stress per se, the pauses and increased articulation time that accompany stress, a combination of these two, or these two plus other influences that improves speech cannot at this time be said. In our experience, however, and for whatever reason, the systematic manipulation of stress is a powerful tool in apraxia of speech treatments.

Constructing and Practicing Contrastive Stress Drills.   To construct a contrastive-stress drill, the clinician need only choose a target, such as a consonant or consonant cluster, and place it in a word. That word can then be set into a sentence made of other words over which the patient has reasonable control. For example, if the patient needs to improve his control of initial /s/, the clinician can put it in a word like "sny," and put "sny" in a sentence such as "Polish the sny." This sentence can then be drilled as a question-answer dialogue. To aid the patient in putting naturally occurring stress on "sny," the clinician asks, "Polish the *what*?" The patient responds "Polish the *sny*." For variety the clinician can ask other questions, thereby causing the primary stress to shift. "Do what to the sny?" "*Polish* the sny." Usually, we begin the drill by having the patient imitate the clinician's equally and evenly stressed production of the utterance before going to the question and answer. This allows the patient to practice with the highest possibility of success and also allows him to memorize the sentence, both of which make success with the rest of the drill more likely. If the patient's more-or-less reflexive use of primary stress in response to a question is insufficient to enhance his articulatory movements, he can be taught to pause longer before the stressed word, or the sentence can be made shorter, or, in some other way, made easier. Any number of sentences containing the target can be practiced; we would usually drill groups of five to ten.

The contrastive-stress drill exploits the facilitating effects of stress and rhythm on articulation, adds variety to treatment, and enhances carryover. Perhaps of greatest importance is the fact that questions and answers are closer to human communication than is the follow-the-leader approach inherent in simple imitation programs.

Combining Gesture and Stress

Combining gestural reorganization and the contrastive-stress drill may be especially powerful. The gestures can slow the utterance, heighten the rhythm and stress profiles, and remind the patient of what he has to do to talk his best. The method is simple. The patient is merely instructed to accompany his answers with gestures. If he has difficulty answering and gesturing, the clinician can model the answer, the gesture, or both, and then systematically provide less and less help. The gesture can accompany each syllable, or selected syllables, and can be faded, or not, as the patient's speech adequacy dictates.

TRANSFER

Control should pass from the clinician to the patient, and improved speech should move from the clinic to the outside. To make these transfers, we use a variety of traditional techniques. We ask questions created to elicit previously practiced words in unpracticed phrases. We then practice these new phrases as a contrastive-stress drill. We have the patient select his own target words and create his own sentences. We have him ask us questions. We engage him in controlled conversations. We have family and others observe treatment. We send work to the ward and to the house. We urge the patient to set aside specific times for practice, and, together with the patient, we set specific goals to be reached outside the clinic. All such activities can be troublesome unless the patient has accepted responsibility for his treatment and has learned to monitor and self-correct. Without them, however, transfer is left in hope's hands, and hope has a notoriously weak grip.

CALLING A HALT

Compensated intelligibility rather than normal speech is the goal of treatment for apraxic speakers; thus the clinician is seldom justified in using normal speech as a criterion for ending treatment. We rely on three indications that treatment should stop. When a patient's system has had enough, it ceases to improve and begins to vary, being sometimes a little better and sometimes a little worse, but being neither good nor bad consistently. The resulting pattern we call a *level sawtooth* and we consider it an important sign that treatment should end. *Failure to generalize* and *failure to maintain* what has previously been learned are the other two signs that an end to treatment is mandatory. The patient whose system treats each stimulus as a new stimulus and each day as a new day deserves to be freed from treatment's rigors. We release such patients to the joys of fishing, walking, or whatever else it was that filled their hours before illness befell them.

REASONS FOR GLEE

Apraxic speakers allow for the best in speech pathology's science and art. If aphasia has not robbed them of understanding, or illness of the will to achieve, they will thrive with appropriate treatment. In our experience, about 90 percent of those patients with an apraxia more severe than their aphasia regain some functional communication. Clinicians can allow themselves to grin when an apraxic talker is referred for treatment.

SELECTED REFERENCES

Fairbanks, G. *Voice and Articulation Drill Book*. New York: Harper and Row, 1960.
Luria, A. *Traumatic Aphasia: Its Syndromes, Psychology, and Treatment*. The Hague: Mouton, 1970.

CHAPTER FIVE

TREATMENT OF FLACCID DYSARTHRIA

Method of Craig W. Linebaugh

Flaccid dysarthria results from involvement of the lower motor neurons, which directly innervate the speech musculature. Thus, neural inputs from intact pyramidal, extrapyramidal, and cerebellar systems are denied the affected muscles because of damage to the "final common pathway." As a result, the denervated muscles of the flaccid dysarthric patient are characterized by hypotonicity or flaccidity, profound weakness, and atrophy.

Denervation also dims the prognosis for the flaccid dysarthric patient. Frequently, too few motor units remain intact to achieve any functional increase in muscle strength and, in turn, the mobility of the affected structures. As a result, flaccid dysarthria demands much of our clinical acumen and resources.

This chapter reflects my conviction that the essential goal for the flaccid dysarthric patient (and, indeed, all whom we serve) must be the most efficient means of communicating he can achieve. To this end, I have devoted most of its content to instrumental techniques for maximizing residual speech intelligibility and compensatory strategies. The reader is referred to the Selected References for more detailed discussions of traditional treatment approaches.

SELECTING AND SEQUENCING TREATMENT OBJECTIVES

The various processes of speech production are inextricably dependent on one another. The order in which we seek to modify these processes must, therefore, be determined on the basis of (1) their relative involvement and (2) their mutual interdependence. For the flaccid dysarthric patient, the first goal should be more efficient use of expiratory air flow. This can best be achieved through improved velopharyngeal closure and respiratory control. Increased vocal fold adduction to decrease air wastage, increased loudness, and improved vocal quality constitute a secondary goal. Improved articulation and prosody remain as final objectives. Note, however, that while full realization of improvement in some processes is dependent on improvement in others, simultaneous attack on various processes is not precluded. Thus, efforts to strengthen the tongue musculature may be undertaken while the patient is being fitted for a palatal prosthesis.

PROCESS-SPECIFIC PROCEDURES

Velopharyngeal Closure/Resonance

Achievement of adequate velopharyngeal closure is critical to the flaccid dysarthric patient, not only for the reduction of hypernasality, but for optimal management of what may be a reduced expiratory air flow and the production of intraoral air pressure for articulation, as well. I employ techniques to improve velar function on a trial basis with all flaccid dysarthric patients with impaired velopharyngeal closure. My primary method incorporates visual feedback of intraoral air pressure.

A polyethelene tube, approximately 5 mm in inside diameter, is placed between the patient's lips. The tube is attached to an air pressure transducer, the output of which is displayed on an oscilloscope. A grid indicating 1 cm H_2O increments of pressure is placed over the screen of the oscilloscope. I instruct the patient "to puff out the cheeks," and model the effect of this gesture on the oscilloscope display. It may be necessary for the clinician, or patient, to manually assist the maintenance of lip closure. The air impounded in the oral and buccal cavities is then released through the nose, and the procedure repeated. Release of the air, nasally, requires opening of the velopharyngeal port and reclosing it for each successive repetition. This procedure is practiced in five sets of ten repetitions each, three to five times during a therapy session. Both the clinician and the patient are provided immediate feedback regarding the patient's performance. The target pressure is gradually increased to a maximum of 10 cm H_2O. I employ this procedure for no more than 10 treatment sessions without an increase to at least 5 cm H_2O of air pressure. When the patient is able to produce 10 cm H_2O of air pressure, or his performance has plateaued above 5 cm H_2O for five sessions, he is turned so that he cannot see the oscilloscope screen, and the procedure is repeated to ensure stable velopharyngeal closure without visual feedback. I consider this weaning procedure a critical step in all of the biofeedback procedures I employ.

Throughout this procedure, and most of those to follow, I direct the patient to attend to the tactile and kinesthetic sensations associated with successful performance of the task. Constant admonitions to "remember that feeling" are provided. This is done in order that the patient may develop a "tactile-kinesthetic template" to serve as both guide and comparator during speech production.

As elegant as the foregoing procedure may appear, the nature of flaccid dysarthria dooms it to failure with oppressing regularity. Thus, I frequently refer patients for a prosthodontic or surgical evaluation. Keep in mind that all patients who have been fitted with a palatal lift prosthesis, or have undergone pharyngoplasty, should receive a period of training. I employ the procedure just described both as a means of obtaining pre-intervention baselines and as a postintervention treatment.

Respiration

Speech production requires essentially no more air than is necessary for sustaining life, but it does require that it be efficiently managed. In particular, the expiratory air flow is to be prolonged and maintained at a relatively constant rate. When the lower motor neurons which innervate the respiratory muscles are affected, this control is diminished.

In order to achieve the controlled expiratory air flow required for speech, I employ a biofeedback procedure similar to that described for velopharyngeal closure. As before, a polyethelene tube attached to a pressure transducer is placed between the patient's lips, and the output of the transducer is displayed on the oscilloscope screen. In addition, a second polyethelene tube, 5 mm in inside diameter and 4 cm long, is also placed between the lips. This tube permits a flow of air from the mouth which approximates that of speech. My experience is consistent with the "5 for 5" rule offered by Netsell and others. Thus, the patient is instructed to maintain a pressure of 5 cm H_2O for 5 seconds. Here, too, the patient is weaned from visual feedback when appropriate, and his attention is focused on tactile and kinesthetic cues related to success.

My other goal with regard to respiration is training in the use of optimal breath groups. Flaccid dysarthric patients, typically, try to produce more syllables on a breath than their other impaired valves can manage effectively. Although the final determination of an optimal number of syllables per breath must await the outcome of treatment directed toward the other processes of speech, I begin training in the planning of shorter breath groups and the appropriate placement of pauses (inspirations) early in the rehabilitation process. This is often a time-consuming goal to reach, and provides a productive interlude between strengthening exercises. Specific activities that I employ include marking prepared passages for appropriate placement of pauses, reformulating long utterances into shorter ones, and describing pictures using several utterances of the desired length rather than fewer long utterances. The objective is to help the patient become accustomed to organizing his linguistic output in units that are manageable by his peripheral speech mechanism. Functional application of this ability is, of course, delayed until training has reached the level at which the patient is expected to produce phase-length units.

Phonation

Weak, breathy phonation indicative of bilateral vocal fold adductor weakness is a common feature of flaccid dysarthria. Resulting from involvement of the X nerves, this impairment of the glottal valve affects the patient's overall speech effectiveness. First, inadequate glottal closure allows the expiratory air flow to pass relatively unimpeded, resulting in inefficient air use and reduced phonation time. Second, reduced glottal resistance results in reduced loudness.

The procedures I employ to improve vocal fold adduction are essentially those of our clinical heritage. Various tension-producing maneuvers (e.g., Froeschel's pushing exercise, pulling up on the bottom of one's chair, pressing the hands together in front of one's chest) are used if the patient has adequate arm strength. Beginning with a "grunt" on release of the tension, the patient is asked to gradually prolong his phonation. The effort applied to the tension technique may be gradually reduced as long as vocal fold adduction is maintained. For patients who require it, the tension maneuver is retained as a facilitatory technique.

Increased loudness comes into play as both a treatment objective and a strategy. The patient sits facing any of a variety of instruments that provide visual feedback regarding intensity of phonation. A microphone is placed directly in front of the mouth. I instruct the patient to produce the loudest sound he can, and then exhort him to produce successively louder sounds on the following repetitions. The vowels /ʌ/ and /æ/ are particularly useful for this procedure. The tension-producing maneuvers already described may be effectively paired with the visual feedback. Again, the patient's attention is focused on developing a tactile-kinesthetic template for increased loudness and vocal fold adduction, and he is systematically weaned from the visual feedback.

Articulation

Involvement of the V, VII, and XII nerves result in impaired movement of the mandible, lips, and tongue, respectively. For the flaccid dysarthric patient, reduced mobility of these structures results in a loss of precision in articulation, which is roughly proportional to the extent of the underlying pathology. Table 1 provides a list of the articulators and the movements required for speech. The muscle groups responsible for each of these movements may be strengthened through exercise. Depending on the degree of weakness, I initially apply assistive force as necessary to achieve a given moment. Later, as strength improves, resistive force may be applied. Exercises are done in five sets of ten repetitions each, three to five times during a therapy session. The patient must also be taught to do these exercises on his own, between sessions. If he is unable to do so, appropriate arrangements should be made for someone to assist him. Five to 10 exercise periods should be conducted daily.

In addition to exercise, I have employed electromyographic (EMG) feedback in strengthening the mandibular musculature. A good electrode placement for mandibular depression is over the anterior belly of the digastricus muscle. For mandibular elevation, an electrode may be placed over the masseter. The integrated EMG activity is displayed on an oscilloscope screen over which has been placed a grid for reference by both the patient and clinician. The

TABLE 1. The articulators and their movements which may require strengthening

Articulator	*Movement*
Mandible	Depression
	Elevation
Lips	Bilabial closure
	Rounding
	Retraction
	Labio-dental approximation
Tongue	Interdental protrusion
	Retraction
	Apical elevation
	Dorsal elevation

patient is instructed to "Clench your teeth/Open your mouth as forcefully as possible." Again the patient's attention is focused on tactile-kinesthetic sensations as successively more forceful contractions are produced.

I have also used EMG feedback to strengthen the labial musculature, particularly the orbicularis oris superior. A surface electrode is placed just lateral to the philtrum, and the patient is instructed to press his lips together as forcefully as possible. A bite block is placed between the molars during this procedure to minimize activity of the mandibular elevators. As before, the integrated EMG activity is displayed on an oscilloscope screen with a reference grid and progressively more forceful target levels are set.

Although considerable attention may be given to strengthening the musculature of the individual articulators, the primary goal remains the most precise articulation that the patient is capable of producing. I approach this at two levels. The first involves work on those specific phonemes or clusters of phonemes with which the patient experiences particular difficulty. The techniques of integral stimulation, phonetic placement, etc. have been well described in the speech pathology literature and need not be reiterated here.

The second level involves the maintenance of adequate articulation for conversational speech. My focus at this level is the determination and maintenance of an optimal articulation rate. Articulation rate refers to the speed of movement of the articulators and is reflected in the duration of individual phonetic segments. Because of weakness of the articulatory muscles, many dysarthric speakers experience slowness of movement and "undershoot" of places of articulation. Undershoot is exacerbated by the patient's use of a faster than optimal articulation rate.

Determination of an optimal articulation rate is accomplished by having the patient repeat phrases at various rates following a clinician model. The fastest rate that yields 95 to 100 percent intelligibility is selected. Simultaneously, the maximum number of syllables the patient can produce comfortably on a breath is determined. At this point, I seek to capitalize on the training in phrasing described earlier. At no time do I ask the patient to produce a phrase longer than this optimal breath group. This would only encourage him to speak at too fast an articulation rate.

Training in maintaining the optimal articulation rate begins with two drills. One involves the patient's repeating phrases at the desired rate following a clinician model. This is done to acclimate the patient to the rate and the sensations associated with it. I have employed DAF at a delay of 50 milliseconds with some patients who had particular difficulty reducing their rate, but this generally is not necessary. I have also required some patients to tap manually as they speak when they were otherwise unable to maintain the desired rate. The second drill involves the patient's making judgments regarding the clinician's rate relative to the desired rate. This is done to focus the patient's attention on rate as a first step in developing self-evaluation skills.

I next require the patient to alter his rate faster or slower in response to my commands, and then in accordance with self-generated commands. This is done to foster the patient's control of his own rate. The patient assesses and records the adequacy of each of his responses. Interjudge reliability between the patient and clinician is checked every 20 utterances. When feasible, the patient practices this drill at home, rating his performance on a score sheet and recording probe lists for clinician evaluation on audio tape. The speech stimuli for these drills are initially a list of 20 to 30 commonly occurring functional phrases. With progress, phrase repetition or reading is replaced by reading of longer passages which is, in turn, replaced by narrative and, then, conversation. At all levels, the patient must evaluate his own performance. When the patient's performance in conversation with the clinician is stable, traditional transfer activities, beginning with the phrases used earlier, are undertaken.

Prosody

Flaccid dysarthric patients generally encounter difficulty achieving stress or natural intonation contours. I have found that loudness is the most readily manipulated factor contributing to prosody for most patients. I generally approach training in altering loudness for stress through contrastive stress drills. I also train patients in the use of pauses to emphasize key words.

AUGMENTATIVE COMMUNICATION SYSTEMS

As noted in the introductory portion of this chapter, the prognosis for achieving intelligible speech is frequently very limited. Thus, a greater proportion of patients with flaccid dysarthria than any other type may require an augmentative communication system. I have equipped and trained patients in the use of a wide variety of augmentative systems, ranging from a simple communicaton board to a specially programmed microcomputer. I have also trained dysarthric patients in the use of Amerind. A discussion of the procedures for selection and training of the use of augmentative communication systems lies well beyond the scope of this chapter, and the reader is referred to the rapidly expanding literature on these systems for specific principles and procedures.

COUNSELING

Anyone familiar with my work knows that I could not complete this chapter without some discussion of counseling. In dealing with flaccid dysarthric patients and their families, I emphasize three essential areas. First, the patient must alter his approach to communication. The successful, efficient transfer of information must be the standard by which all of his communicative attempts are measured. The patient must come to accept "compensated communicative effectiveness" as his goal. This necessitates a change in the patient's self-concept— a self-concept that is already under attack by the dysarthrogenic trauma. Effecting such changes in one's self-concept is nearly always a painful experience and requires skillful counseling and support. I seek to ease this transition by (1) fully explaining the rationale for all that I ask of the patient, (2) making the patient aware of gains in his communicative effectiveness, and above all, (3) always striving for the fastest, most efficient means of communication.

The second area I emphasize is the patient's awareness of listener reaction. In preceding sections, I described in some detail the lengths to which I go to ensure adequate self-evaluation or "internal loop feedback" by the patient. I also train patients to make effective use of "external loop feedback," that is, I train patients to carefully monitor their listeners' reactions (e.g., requests for repetition, facial expression, eye movements, body language). Thus, while internal loop feedback provides the patient information regarding his "physio-acoustic" performance, external-loop feedback provides information regarding his *communicative* performance.

The third area of concern I refer to as "environmental management." Here I discuss and demonstrate for the patient the deleterious effects of various "environmental hazards" to communication. The patient's home environment is analyzed for potential auditory and visual distractors (e.g., television, stereo, dishwasher), and he and his family are made aware of how to best manage them. Floor plans of various sites (e.g., restaurants, stores) are presented and analyzed for the best place to carry on a conversation. Role-playing, with the patient adjusting to his listeners' reactions and managing environmental distractors, is used extensively. I also frequently employ actual field trials as a first step in transferring these skills to the extraclinical environment.

SUMMARY

In dealing with the flaccid dysarthric patient, we must walk the tightrope between prematurely abandoning efforts to improve speech intelligibility, and vainly delaying the implementation of various compensatory or augmentative approaches. In addition, we must deal with the progressive difficulties of those patients with degenerative diseases. Their communicative effectiveness should be monitored at regular intervals, and appropriate intervention provided. This includes not only attention to their speech, but provision or enhancement of augmentative systems in order to maintain maximum efficiency as well.

SELECTED REFERENCES

Darley, F., Aronson, A., and Brown, J. *Motor Speech Disorders*. Philadelphia: W.B. Saunders, 1975.

Johns, D. and Salyer, K. Surgical and prosthetic management of neurogenic speech disorders. In D.F. Johns (Ed.), *Clinical Management of Neurogenic Communicative Disorders*. Boston: Little, Brown and Company, 1978.

Netsell, R., and Daniel, B. Dysarthria in adults: Physiologic approach to rehabilitation. *Archives of Physical Medicine and Rehabilitation*. 1979, *60*:502-508.

Rosenbek, J., and LaPointe, L. The dysarthrias: Description, diagnosis, and treatment. In D.F. Johns (Ed.), *Clinical Management of Neurogenic Communicative Disorders*. Boston: Little, Brown and Company, 1978.

Silverman, F. *Communication Aids for the Speechless*. Englewood Cliffs, N.J.: Prentice-Hall, Inc., 1980.

CHAPTER SIX

TREATMENT OF
SPASTIC DYSARTHRIA

Method of James L. Aten

ANALYZING THE SIGNS

The patient with spastic dysarthria typically reveals significant reductions in the overall intelligibility of speech. After standard testing and recording, I listen for those deviant dimensions that Darley, Aronson, and Brown (1975) report as perceptually characteristic of this type of disorder. Signs commonly noted are a weak, strained-strangled voice, moderate to severe hypernasality, and compromised articulatory movements. These dimensions are then rank-ordered from most to least interfering. The plan for treatment is aimed at reducing or eliminating each aberrant dimension. This chapter presents therapy procedures and rationales I have found effective in modifying the negative influence of the perceived dimensions. The treatment objective, improvement of intelligibility for more adequate social functioning, is attained in the majority of patients who, at onset, have disorders of less severity. Patients with severe disorders reveal slower progress, overall, gain less from treatment, and have frequent periods when they are unintelligible or mute, necessitating use of alternative (nonoral) methods of communication.

CONCEPTUALIZING THE PROBLEMS

Are the signs that we observe in the patient with spastic dysarthria meaningfully different from those noted in other dysarthric patients? Yes, I believe they are. They require an orientation for treatment that begins with certain assumptions about the underlying conditions responsible for these signs. The common denominator is hypertonicity with intended movement throughout the vocal tract. More specifically, the hypertonicity is spastic in nature. This spasticity, unlike that in certain types of rigidity, increases with movement and interferes with coordinated action, creating both an overabundance of tonicity and imbalances in desired ranges of movement. In milder degrees

69

of severity, the onset of spasticity may be gradual, allowing the patient to speak with less impairment in initial words or phrases. With serial movements, as in oral reading, conversation, or prolonged vowels, one observes a reduction in rate, more "weakness" (which may be pseudo-weakness), less air flow, increases in strained-strangled voice quality, and hypernasality. Instrumental documentation of these changes in the literature are limited in number (suggested reading is Smitheran and Hixon, 1981).

I have observed the velum during cineradiography and noted initial elevation followed soon by a progressive failure of the velum to elevate during counting or other serial speech activity. In more severe forms of the disorder, patients reveal an inertia in initiating speech activities. I conceptualize this not as weakness per se, but rather as a rapid onset of increased resistance to stretch. When the latter condition occurs, the patient begins a movement, be it exhalation or vocal fold adduction or tongue-jaw-velar movement that is "nipped in the bud." The result is a poor attempt at evoking the desired movement, as if he were too weak to produce the movement. I believe such patients demonstrate a blocking (rapid onset of spastic contraction) of the movement pattern subserving speech processes.

This conceptualization of the problem leads me to a two-stage recipe for treating the disorder. First, I want all movements to be relaxed and slow to avoid triggering the spastic contractions. Second, I want to shape gradual approximations of full-range movements, retreating to a relaxed baseline whenever spasticity is triggered.

CREATIVE LISTENING

I begin treatment by asking the simple question, "What contributes to this patient's failure to produce understandable speech?" I find that asking this question must often be followed by repeated listening to obtain an answer. I seek to identify an unknown, while predicting an improved level of intelligibility if that dimension (be it hypernasality, strained-strangled voice quality, weak respiratory-phonatory flow, or extreme reduction of oral articulatory movements) were altered. If I listen for a single dimension, I may often fail to assess the gestalt adequately; therefore, I concentrate on "global listening," then predict how the patient would speak if voice, or resonance, or respiration, or articulation were modified toward normal. The answer often provides multiple dimensions of deficit. These "barriers to intelligibility" should then be arranged in a hierarchy. Providing a formula for this is not so simple. I find I sometimes cannot assess the impact of hypernasality on speech until I have obtained a louder voice with sufficient oral pressure to challenge the integrity of velopharyngeal closure. Or, I must encourage more oral movement during maximal effort on the part of the patient to produce the best air (voiced or unvoiced) flow possible, letting hypernasality be constant. What does this have to do with treatment? The answer, in part, is that I find treatment will be more effective and will more readily provide rewards for both the patient and the clinician if we isolate a critical dimension and focus initially on eliminating the negative effect of that characteristic. Netsell (1973) lucidly discusses the point-place system for detecting what levels of speech activities along the vocal tract might be disrupted according to the process or dimension that is deviant. Rosenbek and LaPointe (1978) cogently relate the point-place system to the process model in discussing the obvious overlap between the point-place and process models. The natural and necessary hierarchy of events is: expiration before voice and then oral (and to a far lesser extent nasal) flow as a prerequisite to articulatory production. With reference to severity, I have far less difficulty in deciding what dimension is interfering most with intelligibility in the mild or moderately involved patient. The severe patient may require intervention at the level of respiration to create an audible and briefly sustained phonation before analysis of resonance and articulation. Even then, voice of adequate loudness and duration may be lacking to determine the influence of the nasal and oral "values" on intelligibility. If this is the case, I find I must continue manipulating and enhancing respiratory and phonatory processes before I can realize a firm, valid appraisal of each aberrant dimension.

MORE QUESTIONS PRIOR TO INITIATING TREATMENT

Before launching into application of behavioral methods, I ask the question, "Can the speech processes be medically or prosthetically aided prior to intensive, direct speech therapy intervention?" An analogy may clarify why I feel the need for asking this question. None of us would want to continue speech therapy for the child with an unoperated cleft of the soft palate, if closure of that cleft were imminent and would reduce nasal air flow, and, subsequently, require far less effort and result in more success in speech management. Similarly, medical intervention should be considered for the spastic dysarthric patient. Are there drugs or medications that would elevate the threshold for triggering spasticity? We have tried Dantrium and found that it slightly reduced overall, or at least peripheral, spasticity, but had little or no effect upon speech mechanism musculature. We must keep asking this question, however, because new advances in pharmacology can be anticipated. A more fruitful area currently is prosthetic management. Supporting the abdominal musculature with an elastic band has helped some patients immediately produce better air flow with less effort and reduced strained-strangled phonation, or phonation where none was possible without such girdle assistance. Such intervention may create sufficient voice to continue the listening analysis described previously. Additionally, the use of a reclining wheelchair, or selective posturing in a standard wheelchair, may result in improved vocal production with less effort—consequently, with less contractile interference. Other prosthetic strategies, such as elevating the arms in slings, may allow a patient to initiate and sustain breath with less overall effort when combined with an elastic support or even without such support. Both approaches should be tried in isolation and combination.

Prosthetic intervention utilizing palatal lifts may be helpful in reducing hypernasality. Most of the spastic dysarthric patients have hyperactive gag reflexes. We have fitted a number of these patients at the Long Beach V.A. Medical Center with palatal lifts constructed with flexible twin-wire extensions from the denture acrylic. The lift portion could, therefore, be easily adjusted in the anterior-posterior and vertical planes to allow graduated support to the velum. This approach seems to provide an opportunity to adapt (extinguish partially or completely) the gag reflex to the presence of the lift and gradually tolerate it. An immediate reduction in hypernasality and nasal emission is often noted with less air wastage, improved duration of phonation in some, and some lesser degrees of improvement in articulation precision. The long-range assessment of efficacy from use of palatal lifts with these patients is questionable. In more severe patients, the acute positive benefits appear to dissipate over time, apparently because the velar elevation increases tension in hypopharyngeal and laryngeal musculature after wearing the lift for a few minutes. Patients with less severe disorders do seem to benefit over a longer period of time (assuming hypernasality is a major dimension of their problem) and may not need the lift assistance after a few weeks or months. More careful study of individual patients is needed to determine whether velopharyngeal closure could have been obtained by other means, including gains associated with spontaneous recovery.

A final medical intervention that awaits further investigation is that of surgery, when improvement of voice is found after anesthetizing the recurrent laryngeal and/or superior laryngeal nerves. We are currently initiating work on anesthetizing the laryngeal nerve supply to determine whether a momentary reduction in innervation, unilaterally, will reduce or eliminate the severe spastic dysphonic condition, as Dedo and Shipp (1980) report with spastic dysphonic patients. There may be contraindications (such as deglutition problems) to doing the surgical procedure, but an improvement under anesthesia would offer theoretical support and clinical evidence for increasing our efforts in reducing laryngeal hyperadduction.

REDUCING THE SIGNS

For the sake of organization, I shall discuss procedures aimed at the processes of breathing, phonation, resonation, and articulation in that order, but caution the reader that application must be according to the dictates of the patient's needs, i.e., starting with the most deviant perceptual dimension.

Facilitating Air Flow

I like to establish a breathy sigh by asking the patient to use the *least* amount of breath possible to produce a briefly sustained, relaxed phonation that is audible but essentially voiceless. A few replications of these are all that is necessary in the beginning. The clinician runs the risk of inducing spasticity in obtaining extensive productions before the easy air flow can be shaped to produce voice. Patients may have developed negative breathing patterns with upper thoracic or clavicular tensing and movement, but I deal with this as part of learning a total easy movement pattern. I always try to teach a relaxed sigh by modeling and asking the patient to try to duplicate it before attempting various types of assistance.

If abdominal support is required because the patient cannot self-initiate or prevent overflow tension, I first try a more passive breath release by pushing on the abdominal musculature with both hands. The push should be steady and distribute pressure evenly below the rib cage. Simply, I am trying to support and push the viscera back toward a neutral (resting) position. Patients may be able to create the same type of pressure with their own arm braced against the stomach while stretched across their abdomen, using their hand to grasp the opposite arm of the wheelchair. Patients often need explanations of how to inhale and exhale for economical speech production with demonstrations in, and practice of, correct timing of the pressure and easy release of the exhaled breath stream. I, personally, have not found that providing a bar or braced support for the patient to lean forward against is very successful, as it may signficantly increase overall tension. Finally, some patients do need an elastic wrap (girdle) or other abdominal support. The clinician should be careful not to restrict the lower rib cage. Thoracic restriction disturbs the natural pattern of breathing and may actually induce the upper chest/neck movements, which we seek to eliminate. We have found that a thick leather belt, 2 to 3 inches in diameter, may suffice to offer the necessary support when properly positioned and stabilized around the waist, beneath the ribs.

Reducing Hyperadduction of the Vocal Folds

Stenosis of the laryngeal valve must be reduced or eliminated, if strained-strangled signs are to be ameliorated. Here I have found success with many of the techniques recommended by speech-language pathologists. If we have been successful in obtaining "relaxed" air flow, and elicit a sigh for one or two seconds, the ground work is laid to shape audible phonation that is perceived as less strained or strangled. When initiating therapy at the laryngeal level, the breathy sigh can gradually be shaped into relaxed vowel /a/, or CVC productions that reflect the proper amount of tensing of the vocal folds. I prefer that single-syllable words are begun with the glottal /h/ sound and are followed by open-mouth vowels and a nasal consonant or continuant. I avoid plosives and affricates because of the excess pressure and musculature movement required. Short-duration nasal humming may be needed for some patients to avoid excess contraction of the folds and to feel the balance of easy breath and reduced conscious effort to produce voice. I find that intent (i.e., volitional activity) is often sufficient to trigger muscular spasticity. Severe patients must be encouraged not to force voice but to "let it come." Occasionally, patients seem unable to produce any vocal sound beyond a whispered, or breathy, constricted short utterance. Such patients might benefit from increased effort as Rosenbek and LaPointe (1978) mention, but such effort must not result in excessive overflow of movements and tightness. I only try increasing the effort after I have instructed the patient in relaxed movements that are under control.

Reducing Length of Utterances

Phonatory productions must be kept short. So often, we see patients try to complete their phrases or messages as if they could "beat the onset of the spasticity." It should be pointed out to them that they usually lose this race. They should pause often and repeat those patterns of movements with which they just had success. Nonpropositional conversation, counting, or reading mundane material may facilitate maintaining easy productions.

IMPROVING INTELLIGIBILITY

The patient with spastic dysarthria reveals labored jaw closure, tongue movements that are restricted (particularly isolated velar contacts), and lip closures that, at best, are crude with very limited flexibility. These oral movement deficits, when combined with nasal emission, reduced oral pressure, substitution of voiced for unvoiced consonants, and limited air flow, create a serious articulation sign. I find that initial treatment must usually be directed toward voice onset, serial voice control, and improvement of oral flow by reducing nasal resonance and emission. If these stages of treatment are successful, the foundation has been formed for providing more intelligible speech.

The first objective is to have the patient produce differentiated vowels, beginning with open-mouth vowels /æ/ and /ɑ/ and progressively approximating the higher tongue-jaw vowels /i/ and /u/. Next, I present V-C words or CVCs beginning with /h/. The consonants included, initially, should be continuants or liquids, progressing toward voiced and then unvoiced plosives, leaving the affricates until last. Throughout articulation treatment, I stress the concept of gentle approximation of consonants, emphasizing clear vowel production. Some patients benefit from V-C diphthong combinations such as "I may" or "Oh boy" to reinforce the concept of gliding in a relaxed fashion through consonants with a minimum of constriction and tension. Manipulating the jaw up and down gently to enhance relaxed closure of jaw and lips can be helpful. Later, if tension is under control, I may encourage a more rapid movement of tongue and jaw into, and out of, a closed position to develop approximation of /tʃ/ and /dʒ/ or /k/ and /g/. The patient can be encouraged to assist by head, neck, and body postures, and movements that result in a better acoustic production without excessive increments in tension. Icing may aid initially in reducing tongue retraction and in eliciting a greater range of forward extension.

The overall goal in this process is to achieve a modest improvement in articulatory precision without overflow of tension into the oral or laryngeal/respiratory musculature. Approximation is the key word to symbolize a realistic objective. "Trippingly on the tongue" is not a realistic goal. Abrupt transition and quick articulatory movements only trigger great difficulties a word or two later. We have all experienced the patient who begins on command, "Pʌ-Pʌ-Pʌ," only to have the output shift suddenly to "bʌ-bʌ-bʌ." This tendency can be avoided partially with pausing and gentle movements.

I have had little success, with moderate to severely involved patients, in eliminating monotony or increasing rate. Stress and contrast exercises may be useful toward the end of treatment for the less severe patient. I have not used biofeedback to reinforce relaxation with these types of patients, but I encourage others to so experiment.

ACHIEVING MUSCULAR AND EMOTIONAL BALANCE

As a final guide for treatment, I suggest that nearly every patient with spastic dysarthria can be helped to some degree, if they can achieve a balance between increasing muscular effort without inducing spastic contraction prematurely. Excess effort, or overintention, serves to increase the symptoms and decrease intelligibility. Excess effort and intent increase the likelihood of lability breaks. We find that keeping the patient calm mentally is helpful. Lability can be reduced by systematically teaching the patient to stop and try again and/or to engage in some change of posture or to raise a hand. One such patient was able, using these strategies, to reduce the duration of labile periods from an average of 14 seconds down to four seconds, while also reducing the frequency by 300 percent over a two-week period. Lability is triggered more often in social contexts, and so we have found that group treatment can serve as a medium for desensitizing the patient significantly to social conversational stimuli. Groups also provide an emotionally supportive medium for practicing transfer of skills, and for maintaining skill levels achieved in individual treatment. Generalizations regarding the overall efficacy of treatment are not possible.

SELECTED REFERENCES

Darley, F., Aronson, A., and Brown, J. *Motor Speech Disorders*. Philadelphia: W. B. Saunders Co., 1975.

Dedo, H., and Shipp, T. *Spastic Dysphonia*. Houston: College-Hill Press, 1980.

Netsell, R. Speech Physiology. In F. Minifie, T. Hixon, and F. Willliams (Eds.), *Normal Aspects of Speech, Hearing and Language*. Englewood Cliffs, N.J.: Prentice-Hall, Inc., 1973.

Rosenbek, J., and LaPointe, L. The Dysarthrias: Description, Diagnosis and Treatment. In D. Johns (Ed.), *Clinical Management of Neurogenic Communicative Disorders.* Boston: Little, Brown and Co., 1978.

Smitheran, J., and Hixon, T. A Clinical Method for estimating laryngeal airway resistance during vowel production. *Journal of Speech and Hearing Disorders,* 1981, *46*:138-146.

CHAPTER SEVEN

TREATMENT OF ATAXIC DYSARTHRIA

Method of Thomas Murry

The communicative problems of the ataxic patient evolve from irregular variations in the movements of the desired articulators in the appropriate direction within a normal time period. Thus, the speech and voice characteristics demonstrated by these patients generally include consonant imprecision, improper stress, irregular articulatory breakdown due to dysmetria, past pointing, disdiadokokinesia, tremor, and hypotonia. Since the patient has damage to the cerebellum, his capacity for integrating timing, range, and direction in the precise manner needed for speech is reduced. Although the appropriate systems for initiating speech motor behaviors are present, the degrees to which the desired movements are achieved are highly variable.

The primary goal in the treatment of ataxic dysarthria is to improve overall speech intelligibility to a functional level. Specific treatment should be directed toward improving voice quality and the laryngeal subsystems, increasing articulatory precision, and stabilizing temporal factors associated with rate and appropriate stress of speech. With such a multifaceted problem, the ataxic patient presents a challenge to the therapist to select the proper starting point and, further, to integrate the chronology of treatment for maximum effectiveness. The long-term outcome is often dependent upon the clinician's ability to periodically assess treatment strategies and modify the approach accordingly.

INITIAL ASSESSMENT

Treatment should always include some initial assessment procedure to identify the presence of symptoms, the severity of the problem, and the patient's understanding and awareness of his problem. A neuromoter examination for speech is normally given at the first visit. In addition, an audio recording is made of sustained phonation (usually / i, ɑ, ʊ, æ /), several phrases, reading of a short paragraph, and a few minutes of conversational speech. This allows me to assess the speech characteristics separately from voice characteristics and to make judgments of severity of the phonatory, articulatory, and temporal problems separately. The microstructure of speech (the phonemes and transitions) often provide cues as to the strengths in the macrostructure (spontaneous speech) of the ataxic patient's speech problems. Since rate is often a deviant feature of ataxic speech, a measure of diadochokinesis (pʌ, tʌ, kʌ, etc.) and a timed repetition of a six- or seven-syllable phrase is also useful. Because the main purpose of the assessment is to identify the specific problems of one patient, it is not necessary to compare all measures with normal speakers. Rather, the clinician seeks to classify his patient with respect to other ataxic patients he has treated. Therefore, the actual assessment battery need not come from a standardized test (of which there are really no complete assessment batteries for ataxic dysarthrics), but the clinician should attempt to administer the assessment protocol in the same manner each time.

After making the assessment, I often talk to the patient regarding his motivation and concern for his speech. Those patients whose ataxia is the result of multiple sclerosis are generally motivated, young to middle-aged men who have a strong desire to continue working and, thus, are highly motivated to begin treatment. Once the disease has progressed, the patient is often satisfied with a minor improvement in speech or will refuse treatment due to his awareness of the disease progression. I often point out to these patients that they will always have a need to communicate with family members, doctors, medical staff, and others. Therefore, they should try a course of treatment and attempt to maintain the level at which they are now speaking.

The techniques to be presented are useful in the treatment of ataxia due to cerebellar damage. Friedreich's ataxia, a disease of the cerebellum and brain stem with occasional involvement of the cerebrum, requires additional considerations, and these will be presented at the end of this chapter.

ESTABLISHING A BASE

The problems of the ataxic include a number of voice parameter deficiencies. In order to establish an underlying basis for the treatment of these components, I begin at the level of the respiratory system. By doing so, the patient is able to establish control over the respiratory cycle, which will later be modified by the phonetic and prosodic components of the speech. Three phases can be identified in this treatment: (1) regularity of the respiratory cycle, (2) addition of voicing to the respiratory cycle, and (3) starting and stopping of speech and respiration at appropriate times in the respiratory cycle. A fourth phase, control of prosody, will be dealt with later. These three phases become the building blocks of functional intelligibility.

The ataxic patient is troubled by respiratory irregularity, even in cases of mild ataxia. This is complicated by short or shallow expiration in most cases. It is necessary to have the patient sitting on a chair with both feet on the floor or in a wheelchair in which the feet reach the floor or the footrests. The patient begins by simply practicing exhalation at a steady rate on cues from the clinician. After showing the patient what to do, I ask him to produce exhalations 3 to 4 seconds in length. Steady exhalation is the goal. Once this is reached, a rhythm paradigm is established with inhalation, 3 to 4 seconds of exhalation, 2 to 3 seconds of rest, and then a repetition of the process. The basic procedure is often augmented by having the patient place an open hand over the abdominal area (without pressure) or by having him use a slight glottal frication during exhalation. This helps to reduce the flow of air and thus improve the patient's chances of prolonging the flow to 4 seconds. There is no reason to demand extra-long expiratory cycles. Assuming a flow rate of approximately 200 cubic centimeters of air per second (cc/sec.), 3 to 4 seconds of exhalation would use about 1½ times the adult male tidal volume. There is rarely a need to establish control of the expiratory cycle beyond this level for most speaking situations.

Once I establish a reasonable steady tidal respiratory cycle, I add voicing. Initially, the patient is asked to add a steady voice to the expiratory cycle. The clinician must be aware of explosive bursts as well as interruptions in the voice signal. I use the /ɑ/ and the /i/ vowels for this step. If initiation is difficult or interrupted, I ask the patient to use a fricative such as /f/ or /h/ so that he may hear the flow of air first, followed by the vocalic portion.

Since sensory monitoring is useful in this type of treatment, it may be helpful to the patient to view some type of meter during his steady phonations. In my experience, I have found that the most useful devices are the simplest so as not to distract the patient from the basic work of steady expiratory air flow during tidal volume. This treatment is continued until the patient can maintain a steady vocal output for 3 to 5 seconds.

The next step is to initiate simple, but useful, one-syllable words on the steady expiratory cycle. Words such as *hi, bye, yes, no, me, I, you, where, when, who,* etc. are practiced until the patient can produce each on a cue from the therapist without an explosive onset or interruption. Since this drill is directed at controlling respiration, little attention is paid to voice quality at this time.

The third stage of the basic respiratory treatment is directed toward producing several syllables on one expiration. In this phase, the patient begins to approximate the normal rhythms of speech. At first, the only demand is to produce several syllables on one expiratory cycle. For example, he may be asked to say ba, ba, ba on one breath with a discrete pause between syllables. If this phoneme combination is too difficult, I start with ha, ha, ha. Eventually, the level of difficulty is increased to such things as counting to three, combining syllables, as in basketball game, in which there is only one pause in the expiratory cycle (after basketball), and the phrase becomes intelligible.

It is necessary to progress beyond three syllables on one expiratory cycle, but this should be done only when the patient has good control over the on-off laryngeal/respiratory mechanisms for three or less syllables. It is not surprising to find that progression beyond three syllables is difficult, especially if phonetic content is not controlled. Again, I start with simple phrases such as a pa pa pa. This allows the patient to monitor the respiratory activity while paying little attention to meaning. At this point in treatment, I am not concerned about the stress patterns of the phrases; rather, I am primarily interested in seeing that the patient can stop and start the respiratory/vocal systems in a controlled manner.

VOICE

The voice of the ataxic patient has been described as having a harsh component as well as a tendency toward monotone and monoloudness. I have found these vocal attributes to be present in the ataxic, but, in addition, I have noted several other pitch aberrations. Specifically, vocal pitch often exceeds normal pitch changes on interrogative statements. Also, the ataxic may drop his pitch inordinately low in attempting a long utterance. This low pitch, which may be vocal fry, is often mistaken for some type of "harshness." Loudness also shows extreme fluctuation, especially if the patient lacks controls of his respiratory musculature. This is seen as a loud first syllable followed by a soft voice for the remainder of the expiratory cycle.

Since the use of the voice is so important, not only to vowel quality and separation of cognate pairs, but also to proper use of word stress, I spend considerable time in voice drills. Pitch change, an important parameter of syllable and word stress, is often an easy task for the patient. It also reinforces control of the respiratory system. I do not attempt to change the overall pitch of the voice. Rather, I feel it is important to inject the proper pitch contour into the meaning of the message. Thus, pitch variation drills dovetail with treatment of stress.

I begin with several basic three- or four-syllable models such as: *It's a nice day. How are you? Is that it! What time is it? It's time to go.* Once I hear how the patient says these phrases, I use either pitch increases or decreases to specify a meaning. In the case of extreme pitch fluctuations, I attempt to "smooth" the pitch contour. This is done with visual aids such as a grease pencil on a mirror or standard pen and paper. I draw the pitch pattern that the patient presents along with the desired pattern. Initially, I try to stay away from big variations in pitch and progress toward increased pitch variation.

For the ataxic patient whose pitch usage gives the impression of drunkenness, the pitch drills must be directed on the initial syllable or two, which often have great peaks or troughs. This is similar to the way a record sounds if you put the needle on the groove first and then start it up. For these patients, it may be necessary to drill with simple consonant-vowel (CV) syllables just to establish steadiness of pitch at the onset. Exercises for reducing strain and constriction of the laryngeal musculature presented in other chapters of this volume may be useful for these patients. Once the initial syllable can be produced with some pitch control, the work moves quickly to the control of pitch over an expiratory cycle.

When the pitch changes have been brought under control by either increasing or decreasing pitch variations as necessary, exercises in which therapist and patient interact in a conversational mode may be tried. I like to write out the possible responses that the patient will give so that he can plan his pitch usage. If that is successful, we deviate from the prepared script. It doesn't hurt to keep drawings of pitch contours available so that the patient may refer to them for his responses.

A word of caution about pitch drills. I try to stay within the normal expiratory cycle for all pitch drills. This means they are confined to a duration of about 3 to 5 seconds. Also, it is best to avoid sing-song patterns at the syllable level, since these have little relationship to normal intonation usage. For therapists who feel that they have a "tin ear," it may be wise to limit pitch variation drills to simple rising-falling or steady contours. However, I have noted that even clinicians who profess complete pitch indiscrimination can be trained to identify simple contours.

Another vocal feature in the ataxic is "harshness or hoarseness" (I generally refer to this quality as "roughness," since it reflects aperiodicity in the vocal output). This quality may derive from abnormal adjustments in muscle contraction, causing too much or too little muscle contraction, or contraction of the improper muscles when attempting to initiate or change a vocal dimension. Certainly, treatment already described will reduce some of the laryngeal tension associated with improper breathing. Other exercises should seek to initiate voicing at some "mid-level," that is, not at the extremes of pitch or loudness. Visual observations of the neck and facial musculature is often a cue to the patient as to the amount of force being generated at the onset of phonation. Postural considerations, such as hyperextended chin or "hunching" while seated, may also contribute to rough voice quality. Keep the chin tucked in and parallel with the floor.

Loudness problems in the ataxic generally stem from inability to control specific features of the speech signal such as stress and voice onset. When respiration is controlled and stress is used properly, loudness aberrations diminish. However, drills that make use of a VU meter, or loudness contours drawn on paper, may be useful. This is especially true if the patient is having difficulty with pitch-changing exercises. The loudness problems are often more than monoloudness. Rarely will I work on loudness alone as I might do in a patient having a hyperfunctional voice disorder. Rather, I use multisyllabic words and phrases to effect a planned loudness pattern that is consistent with breath group usage. For example, with the phrase, *How are you?*, I might suggest increasing loudness on one word such as: *How ARE you?* An alternative production might be: *How are YOU?* Conversely, most of us would not consider increasing loudness on the first word, *HOW*. But in the phrase, *Who are you?* *WHO* may also be emphasized with increased loudness.

Drills in the pitch and loudness changes are carried out until the patient is able to select one or the other parameter and vary it, in order to change the meaning or emphasize the desired word. Conversation or oral reading may be suggested to augment the voice exercises.

ARTICULATION

Articulatory deficiencies in ataxia include not only consonant imprecision, but also distortion of vowels. The severe articulation disturbances derive from the ataxic's inability to control the range of movement and timing patterns of the lips, tongue, and jaw. With the ataxic patient, there is no substitute for intensive phoneme drill, first using isolated consonants and then blending them into speech patterns. Since the ataxic is generally slow in these movements, it is important to conduct articulatory drills at a moderate rate somewhat faster than the patient's general rate of speaking. I usually progress from sounds that are moderately distorted to severely distorted ones. Movement and rhythm should be emphasized in the single consonant drills.

As the patient acquires facility with the basic articulation movements of single consonants, the drills are incorporated into syllables with the vowels /a,i,u/. These vowels are used since they represent the extremes of tongue height and tongue advancement. A sequence of drills might consist of the following:

/ pi, pi, pi, pi, pi, pi, pi, pi, pi /
/ pɑ, pɑ, pɑ, pɑ, pɑ, pɑ, pɑ, pɑ, pɑ /
/ pu, pu, pu, pu, pu, pu, pu, pu, pu /
/ pi, pi, pi, pi, pi, pi, pi, pi, pi /
/ ti, ti, ti, ti, ti, ti, ti, ti, ti /
/ tɑ, tɑ, tɑ, tɑ, tɑ, tɑ, tɑ, tɑ, tɑ /
/ tu, tu, tu, tu, tu, tu, tu, tu, tu /
/ ti, tɑ, ti, tɑ, ti, tɑ, ti, tɑ, ti /
/ pi, ti, pi, ti, pi, ti, pi, ti, pi /

This progression would continue until the three vowels and two consonants were combined in all contexts. Gradually, the voicing contrast (/pi, bi/) would be introduced. This would be followed with word and phrase drills such as:

/ pip, pɑp, pip, pɑp . . . . /
/ tit, tɑt, tit, tɑt . . . . /
/ pɑp tɑt pit; tik tɑp tuk . . . . /

In these drills, consonant precision, vowel color, and rhythm are all considered. When the patient is severely unintelligible, the phoneme drill must focus on one or two phonemes at a time; such things as vowel distortion and rhythm must be sacrificed initially until the patient achieves success in the movement to and from the point of articulation. I work with exaggerated movements early, but try to keep a rhythm to the movements. Since the ataxic may show irregularities in his articulation, a rhythm pattern is often helpful to regulate the sequencing from phoneme to phoneme. Tapping while talking is useful in establishing a rhythm pattern. Usually, I tap first to establish a moderate rate. If the patient can acquire a metronomic sense in these early drills, intelligibility improves in conversational speech even if he never achieves normalized temporal patterns. We must not forget that our goal is useful, intelligible speech. Precision of consonant production is an essential contributor to intelligibility.

In the diagnostic and periodic assessments I make of ataxic patients, I have noted a feature, which might be called "target velocity," that appears to be highly related to consonant precision. Target velocity refers to the speed utilized in reaching the point of articulation, and then continuing on, through and away from the target once it has been reached. The target velocities of the ataxic are slow and often complicated either by not reaching the point or by delay in moving away from the point. This is especially true in plosive consonants. Some individuals will remain at the point of lip closure (for/p/) or tongue-palate contact (for/t/) as long as three times that of the normal talker. Thus, the reason I try to set a rhythm to all articulation drills is to get the patient not only to reach the desired point, but also to continue through the movement. Word repetition in which no two adjoining phonemes are the same (e.g., *cup, top, thick, shape*) provide a good drill to increase normal target velocity. Of course, phrases that are meaningful are more interesting to the patient (*Pass the dish, please*).

The patient with cerebellar disease has a hypotonic pattern of articulation. That is, the musculature lacks the tonus to function accurately. I feel that considerable time must be spent in working at various articulatory rates without sacrificing precision. If the patient can control target velocity at various rates, he has learned compensatory coarticulation patterns sufficiently to use them in conversational speech.

I like to use a mirror when doing vowel drills. Since most vowels have visible features such as lip rounding, lip protrusion, and jaw opening, I use sustained vowel drills in front of a mirror to focus attention on both the auditory and visual picture each vowel presents. Again, exaggerated movements are helpful in the beginning. Then, drills involving moderately rapid movements from one vowel position to another following a prescribed metric are used to counteract the hypotonia. Since range of movement is reduced in hypotonia, vowel, vowel-consonant, and consonant-vowel combinations must be chosen to maximize the movement of articulators. Drills with vowels only, such as / i_____ ɑ_____ i_____ ɑ_____ / and / i_____ u_____ i_____ u_____/, are helpful and can be done by the patient at home. Vowel-consonant-vowel drills emphasize the movement toward the consonant and back toward a prescribed vowel. I have presented the idea that compensation for hypotonia and target velocity are integral features of the ataxic's articulatory skills. We will see shortly how they also relate to prosodic skills. However, it is important to focus on the precision of phoneme production when doing articulation drills. These drills are intended to improve articulation and not to substitute for prosodic therapy. I try to ignore the dysrhythmias at first, concentrating on articulatory precision and target velocity. I like to listen to tape-recorded articulatory drills. These help me to focus on the sounds that need additional treatment as well as those that have appropriate target velocities. The latter can then be reinforced in a variety of metrics, while the former are given additional time to achieve articulatory precision.

PROSODIC ASPECTS

From the foregoing discussion of the ataxics' problems, it is obvious that poor timing and improper use of word stress interfere with all components of speech output. At this stage of therapy, we are achieving two important functions: improved intelligibility and increased acceptability. To do this, three aspects of prosody must be treated: (1) the slow rate already alluded to; (2) proper timing of individual sounds, which I referred to in the preceding section; and (3) stress and intonation. Appropriate use of stress has a direct affect on acceptability of the ataxic's speech. I like to use three or four syllable phrases to begin this treatment, for example, *Baseball is fun*. In this phrase, we try to achieve emphasis on the first syllable of *baseball* and, also, avoid a pause or break between the two syllables in the word. With the proper respiratory training, there would be no need to completely stop the expiratory cycle except for the very brief time it takes to articulate the plosives. If this phrase is difficult, we might change to one in which there are no plosives or the plosives are only at the beginning or end of the phrase (e.g., *Silver is soft; Come over for lunch*). If the patient maintains the expiratory flow, he will avoid the pulsatile character so often seen in ataxia, that is, the ataxic might say: *Sil ____ ver ____ is ____ soft* (I have used spacing to indicate a temporal distortion). This pulsing has been called "scanning" or "measured speech," and refers to the equal stress applied to each syllable along with the lengthening of intervals between words and syllables. To treat this problem, I refer back to early music lessons in which we were taught to create a phrase out of single notes to tell the "story" with meaning. The ataxic must therefore use his respiratory system to govern the outward flow of air while combining syllables within each phrase. At first, this is done slowly, but then the rate is increased. A slow rate of speaking, when phrased properly, is more acceptable (and often more intelligible) than a faster rate in which there are pauses between every syllable and the speech takes on a "staccato" character.

In the early syllable drills, I review tape recordings to determine whether the patient is using pitch, loudness, timing, or a combination of these to create the appropriate prosody. However, before working on one specific prosodic feature, I spend a great deal of time on connected phrasing. Once the patient learns to produce a phrase on an expiratory cycle without interrupting each word or syllable, I then use either pitch or loudness to add to the prosodic control. Feedback is useful especially to maintain the overall rate of speaking. I have found that a two-channel oscilloscope helps. On one channel, I put the desired pattern; the patient tries to match this pattern on the second channel. For strictly pitch-related prosody drills, the Language Master or a similar device is useful.

FRIEDREICH'S ATAXIA

Friedreich's ataxia is neurologically quite different from cerebellar ataxia due to involvement of the spinocerebellar tracts. In addition to the previous discussion of cerebellar patients, other dysarthric chacteristics must be treated in patients with Friedreich's ataxia. I find that this patient typically has more explosive speech than the cerebellar ataxic. In addition, the phonatory characteristics are more bizarre in that there is a rough, or harsh, quality along with a strained-strangled quality.

Treatment of this group focuses on respiratory/phonatory aspects of speech. Intelligibility can be improved by controlling the explosive release at the onset of phonation. After basic respiratory training, I begin with easy interrupted phonation such as / i_____ i_____ i_ i_____/. This is then modified to add fricative consonants: /fi_____ fi_____ fi_____ fi_____/ and then plosive consonants: /bi_____ bi_____ bi_____ bi_____/. If the patient can accomplish these simple phonatory/articulatory movements, I increase the complexity. Since onset is important, training in awareness of the respiratory air cycle is necessary. If the voice is exploded, the patient must interrupt the exercise and begin again. Use of nasals or liquids often helps to "defuse" the plosiveness of the ataxic's speech.

There is a tendency for the patient with Friedreich's ataxia to increase pitch. I try to set a pitch level for the drills and maintain it as the complexity increases. This helps to reduce pitch breaks into falsetto, as well as aphonia. Also, too high a pitch tends toward a more strained-strangled quality, whereas too low a pitch leads to the perception of a rough voice quality.

COMMENT

Treatment of patients with neuromotor speech disorders is often limited, owing to intervening neurological sequelae, a general regressive condition, or factors relating to age. The therapist has little or no control over these. However, by regular assessments, expansion of basic treatment protocols to include daily living functions, and treatment modules that are generally successful to the patient in terms of increased intelligibility, the therapist becomes a positive force in the patient's life. When intelligibility is functional and neuromotor speech assessments indicate a plateau, the therapist must prepare to discontinue treatment. Unless close control is kept of the progress or lack of progress, both the patient and the therapist will experience an investment of time with decreasing returns, frustration, and frequent cancellations. Treatment should be terminated on a positive basis. Patients should be encouraged to continue drills in order to maintain functional intelligibility.

REFERENCES

Berry, W. and Goshorn, E. Oscilloscopic feedback in the treatment of ataxic dysarthria. American Speech-Language-Hearing Association Convention, Atlanta, Georgia, 1979.

Darley, F., Aronson, A., and Brown, J. *Motor Speech Disorders*. Philadelphia: W. B. Saunders Co., 1975.

Kent, R. and Netsell, R. A case study of an ataxic dysarthric: Cineradiographic and spectrographic observations. *Journal of Speech and Hearing Disorders,* 1975, *40*:115-134.

Kent, R., Netsell, R., and Abbs, J. Acoustic characteristics of dysarthria associated with cerebellar disease. *Journal of Speech and Hearing Research,* 1979, *22*:627-648.

Rosenbeck, J. and LaPointe, L. The dysarthrias: Description, diagnosis and treatment. In D. Johns (Ed.), *Clinical Management of Neurogenic Communicative Disorders*. Boston: Little, Brown and Co., 1978.

Yorkston, K. and Beukelman, D. Ataxic dysarthria: Treatment sequences based on intelligibility and prosodic considerations. *Journal of Speech and Hearing Disorders,* 1981, *46*:398-404.

CHAPTER EIGHT

TREATMENT OF HYPOKINETIC DYSARTHRIA

Method of Bill Berry

Hypokinetic dysarthria is not uncommon. It generally results from parkinsonism, although it has been reported in Wilson's disease, in progressive supranuclear palsy, and in patients who are being treated by large doses of psychotropic medication. In these conditions, the primary neurologic disorder is treated medically, usually with drug management. When hypokinetic dysarthria is involved, the speech clinician can provide a series of valuable services: evaluation, treatment, and education.

EVALUATION SERVICES

The great majority, probably more than 98 percent, of patients suffering from hypokinetic dysarthria referred to a speech pathologist have Parkinson's disease, a relatively common degenerative condition. It is important for the speech clinician to have a good understanding of the general course of this disease or any of the others that cause this dysarthria. I must be conversant with the referral physician about the neurologic symptomatology, the neurophysiologic mechanisms involved, as well as the various medical/surgical treatments and their prognosis. It is quite logical for a physician to hesitate to refer patients with dysarthria to me if I do not understand their medical problems. I find it necessary to have a basic understanding of parkinsonism, to know how to evaluate an adult with dysarthria, and to know how to differentiate hypokinetic dysarthria from other symptom categories such as ataxic, flaccid, spastic, hyperkinetic, or mixed.

It is very important to obtain carefully controlled audiorecordings and pertinent acoustic/physiologic data prior to, and at selected intervals during, treatment. In this way, reliable data can be generated to reflect the effects of drug management, behavioral therapy, environmental education, and/or time. The latter, of course, is a significant variable in diseases that, like parkinsonism, are degenerative.

91

It has been my experience that referring physicians often question the role of a "speech therapist" when their patient's speech is getting worse. However, they do not hesitate to refer when they realize that it is also my role to document the degenerative process, to continually re-evaluate the communicative problems reported by the patient, and to educate/counsel with the patient and others about what they might be doing to counteract these problems. Therefore, the evaluation methods, the character of the resulting data, as well as the pertinence of the evaluation reports (initial/progress) may be important factors if I am attempting to cultivate dysarthria referrals, but am not getting results.

Generally, after having initially evaluated a patient with hypokinetic dysarthria in whom intelligibility is moderately-to-severely reduced, the patient's speech will be characterized by reduced prosodic variability (i.e., monotony), accelerated rate (often short rushes of speech with prolonged interphrase pauses), reduced loudness, breathy phonation, and reduced articulatory excursion. Therefore, it is not difficult to understand why individuals with more chronic Parkinson's disease report difficulty in being understood over the phone, in group conversations, in noisy places, or by individuals who are not accustomed to the patient's speech. These complaints are certainly not unique to the individual with hypokinetic dysarthria. Yet, the intensity and character of these problems must be handled individually and the pattern of management decisions will, therefore, be unique for each patient.

TREATMENT SERVICES

Prophylactic Management

Diagnosis of Parkinson's disease is often made when there is no dysarthria. If practical to do so, and lines of professional communication are established, I prefer that the patient be referred at this point. Early referral to a speech clinician is advantageous for several reasons.

First, it allows the clinician to gather baseline speech data before dysarthria is a problem. These data can later be used for comparison and documentation when speech complaints become apparent. This initial evaluation also provides the opportunity to begin education about dysarthria (all patients with parkinsonism ultimately suffer from hypokinetic dysarthria). If I were the patient, I would want to know what my clinician knows so that I would have more control over my future.

This leads to the issue of prophylaxis. Actually, I am overstating the case to imply that I could treat the patient early in the disease and "prevent" hypokinetic dysarthria. My goal would rather be to impede the degenerative process. Through a directed exercise program designed to promote increased breath support, increased range of motion of articulators, exaggerated prosodic variability, and reduced speech rate, the hypothesis could be presented that a motivated patient could decrease the effects that increased muscle rigidity and decreased rate control have on the speech mechanism in chronic hypokinetic dysarthria. This involves:

1. Use of traditional inspiratory/expiratory exercises to promote maximal vital capacity in respiration.

2. Use of exaggerated chewing and equally exaggerated slow alternate motion rate tasks to achieve maximal range of motion in articulation.

3. Carrying this over into sentence repetition and question/ drills where the patient markedly overemphasizes stress and melody changes.

4. Utilizing behavioral modification techniques to reduce the rate of speech while the patient still has the ability to do so.

Here, you will be working with a normal speaker, or possibly a mildly dysarthric individual, to educate and motivate change in habit patterns while he has the neuromuscular capacity. Later, if and when a patient reaches the stage when most referrals are made, the aforementioned behavioral techniques generally produce minimal results. For years, physical therapists have been encouraging patients with parkinsonism to squeeze rubber balls and do range-of-motion exercises, including exaggerated facial expressions, to counteract the degenerative processes. It takes early referral, perseverance, and self-motivation but it helps. Early referral is the key to this process.

Drug Management

Now let us get more realistic. The treatment that is likely to have the most positive physical effects on an individual with Parkinson's disease is drug management. Since the neurologist or referring physician will be the team leader in this treatment, here we have a selling point for a carefully documented speech evaluation, performed before, and at selected intervals during, the treatment. Neurologists are most receptive when they learn that you can provide extremely reliable data such as: (1) alternate motion rate of syllable repetition, (2) relative speech intensity (range/averages), (3) range of vowel fundamental frequency variability, and (4) pausetime, vowel duration, and other speech rate measures. All of these objective measures can be obtained oscillographically from carefully standardized, acoustically controlled audiotape recordings. This, of course, requires specialized equipment and the ability to use it. Technology should be our ally, not a burden. Many clinics are capable of providing sophisticated physiologic speech measures that would certainly be pertinent. All of these are data points that can help the neurologist to determine the effects of drug management and help me to decide whether any significant changes have taken place in the speech of our patients with hypokinetic dysarthria.

Behavioral Management

The number of therapy suggestions in this section will be directly proportional to my success in speech therapy with patients suffering from chronic, severe hypokinetic dysarthria. Unfortunately, most who suffer from parkinsonism are not referred to speech clinicians until the degenerative process is well advanced, leading to significant intelligibility problems. It has been my experience that few of these individuals respond significantly to behavioral treatment. Generally, in chronic Parkinson's disease, progress is minimal, and this severely challenges the motivation of most patients. We are asking our patient to fight upstream against the currents of increasing muscular rigidity. With many it takes personal commitment, a great deal of time (which can mean many dollars), and social sacrifices to do the behavioral exercises that will yield only minimal gains in intelligibility.

Reading this, you may ask, "Then why do therapy at all?" I firmly believe that this is a question that must be confronted by the patient as well as the clinician. The patient should be informed of the prognosis for success, and a realistic definition of success should be at the heart of this information. If, then, the patient chooses to forge ahead, here are some practical points that should be pursued.

Neuromuscular rigidity is the reason for hypokinetic dysarthria. This affects the respiratory system (reduced loudness), the laryngeal mechanism (breathiness), the upper airway system (reduced articulatory excursion), as well as the prosodic output of speech (monotony, short rushes, rapid rate). All of these are factors that produce the intelligibility problems experienced by the patient. With this in mind, every possible action should be taken to increase the general physical activity level of the patient, to impede secondary postural changes, such as contractures or stooping, and to promote good muscle tone. Therefore, I cooperate with the dietician and the physical therapist to develop a program of proper diet and exercise. Obesity reduces breath support for speech which, of course, is already a problem in parkinsonism. Sedentary physical habits reduce muscle tone and produce orthopedic contractures, making it all the more difficult for the hypokinetic patient to initiate speech, to control rate, and to speak loudly enough. Inactivity from depression and withdrawal is an insidious whirlpool that many parkinsonian patients get caught in and cannot get out of without help. So I reach in and help pull the patient out; I get them on a regular home exercise program in graduated steps; I work to achieve maximal sitting and/or standing postures for speaking; and I get the patient's weight to an optimum level. All of these things will provide signs of motivation and the foundation for whatever progress can be expected. If none can be achieved, to be candid, speech therapy efforts are likely to be fruitless.

If the patient responds to this program and I slowly begin to integrate speech drills into the patient's regimen of activities, I get the most out of them. I concentrate on rate control. Forget the temptation toward traditional articulation therapy. Hypokinetic dysarthrics generally do not distort phonemes in the manner that characterizes other types of dysarthria. Therefore, "good ole artic therapy" simply will not pay dividends. The patient must learn to turn a mental key and slow the rate of speech when there is a need to increase intelligibility. He must further learn to reduce the number of polysyllabic, low-frequency words, which are harder to produce and more difficult for the listener to understand. I try to teach my patients to use contextual "starters" when they are on the phone, in groups, or in noisy places. By contextual starters, I mean general semantic cues that are given any time they want to change subjects or speak in abstraction. For example, on the phone my patient learns to say "Let's talk about . . . (pause) . . . baseball" slowly, when he wants to shift to this general topic. The listener is then prepared to listen, and the patient is more likely to remember to concentrate on rate control when the subject matter is announced.

Here are some key points to remember about rate control therapy:

1. Don't expect your patient to learn to slow rate 100 percent

of the time. I use a mental "key" image and tell the patient to "turn the key" only when he needs to increase intelligibility.

2. Concentrate on short phrases or single word responses whenever possible. The longer the patient with hypokinetic dysarthria talks, the more likely he is to lapse into rapid, short rushes of speech.

3. External feedback techniques can be helpful. Delayed auditory feedback (DAF) is used to promote kinesthetic awareness of slower rate, but DAF used only in therapy has not been shown to have carry-over value into spontaneous speech. I will comment later about portable DAF. External visual cues—subtle gestures like a raised finger or a wink—can be used by the clinician, and later taught to family members to signal to the patient that he must concentrate more on slowing rate.

4. A visual feedback system, by which amplified/filtered speech can be displayed oscilloscopically to the patient immediately following a spontaneous or repeated response, is encouraged as a therapy tool. This technique can be very helpful in giving the patient an extrasensory channel to monitor speech while rate control skills are being learned.

5. Finally, measure speech at appropriate intervals. You are hypothesizing that the patient can learn to slow his rate, or that he must eliminate aphonic episodes, or that intensity should be increased to promote an increase in intelligibility. Therefore, you should be measuring variables that can tell you whether the patient is achieving intelligibility, word or phrase duration, or speech intensity objectives. One recently published source that I feel has great promise is the *Assessment of Intelligibility of Dysarthric Speech* by Yorkston and Beukelman (1981). If your data are positive, forge ahead. If, however, progress is not realized, time and money will be wasted by proceeding, and another approach, such as portable DAF, might be more productive.

Electroprosthetic Management

Electroprosthetic management is a fancy term for portable DAF, a device that was developed with the hypokinetic dysarthric in mind. Hanson and Metter (1980, 1982) described its use and success, and it may have promise. We have known for many years that patients with parkinsonism can slow their rate of speech and be more intelligible under the effects of DAF. Until recently, however, DAF was produced by using large audiotape recorders. Now, DAF units are being produced commercially in a size that makes them portable. The cost is approximately $800, and the only manufacturer I know of prefers to deal through clinics and offers a 30-day trial period. When the device works, as in the Hanson and Metter reports, the results can be remarkable. Though the reduced prosody (i.e., monotony) remains, rate of speech is significantly slower and may be louder, making the patient much more intelligible. However, if this approach is not successful following unsuccessful speech therapy, I come to my "ace in the hole"—the universal management approach.

EDUCATION SERVICES

Environmental education is a universal management approach because it can be utilized with all individuals who suffer from dysarthria (Berry and Sanders, 1982). However, I have encountered dysarthric adults who have never been told that eye contact is important to promote intelligibility. My rule of thumb has become, "Don't assume that your patient is an expert communicator." Carrying this one step further, it is reasonable to assume that the significant others who will be listening to your patient are also less than expert communicators. My hypothesis, therefore, becomes: If my patient and his/her listeners can learn to manipulate selected variables related to verbal interaction, increased intelligibility will result.

This is not a novel approach to communication rehabilitation. Our audiology colleagues call it aural rehabilitation and have been using this educational approach for years to integrate deaf/hard-of-hearing individuals into the verbal world. Therefore, consider almost everything that you have learned about aural rehabilitation; reverse it, and it applies to the adult with dysarthria. I often conceptualize the verbal interaction process with each of us being sender/receivers who must transmit our messages through a series of environmental "filters and/or amplifiers" that can be selectively varied to alter the intelligibility of the verbalization. Think of it. You are the sender, I'm the receiver. You speak, I listen, and we can alter a number of environmental factors to ensure the reliability of the message transfer. Here are some of the variables.

AMBIENT NOISE
LIGHTING
DISTANCE
RESONANCE
POSTURE
SITUATION
EXTERNAL AIDS

If you refer to this conceptual model, a large number of extremely practical suggestions that are often given to the hard-of-hearing can be reversed and can become helpful to dysarthric patients and their listeners. Here are a few examples:

1. Avoid noisy places if you need to be understood.
2. Get as close to your listener as possible.
3. Be sure to look at your dysarthric spouse when he/she is speaking.
4. Get a remote audio control for the TV/radio. Turn it down to call attention to the fact that you want to speak etc. I think you can see that when any of the so-called "filters or amplifiers" in the aforementioned model are altered to favor the dysarthric, intelligibility will be increased. We simply cannot assume that our patients will automatically adjust and learn that they must achieve better eye contact to promote listener speech reading; that they will learn to move closer to their listener; that they will move to a quieter spot in the room to repeat a message; or that they will use special draperies and wall coverings to dampen ambient noise in their homes.

Therefore, from the outset of patient management, information should be provided that could ultimately promote verbal interaction with the patient. Admittedly, the effect of this approach is difficult to measure. A survey or periodic interview allows me to determine whether any of my suggestions are being implemented. Positive subjective reports about the patient's feelings concerning communication may also be evidence that the education is working. However, I do not assume that patients know these things and will make the necessary adjustments. Remember, parkinsonism may be making the patient more rigid. She may have been referred in a chronic, severe state of dysarthria, and the prognosis for any positive results from speech therapy or DAF may be guarded. But environmental education could still help to bring a withdrawn patient out of his/her shell.

In summary:

1. I try to promote early referral from neurologists, who often see patients with parkinsonism before they are dysarthric.
2. I am systematic and as objective as possible in evaluating patients at regular intervals during treatment.
3. I am realistic in treatment goals, especially considering the fact that parkinsonism is a degenerative neurologic disease.
4. I consider environmental education as a universal treatment

approach that could have positive effects on intelligibility and verbal interaction, even when speech therapy might fail. I do not assume that the patient will adjust automatically.

5.   The information that I can provide, the therapy, and/or the team interaction with others treating the patient could ultimately give the patient more control over his/her destiny.

If for no other reason, the latter is justification for intervention with any dysarthric adult.

SELECTED REFERENCES

Berry, W., and Sanders, S. Environmental Education: The universal management approach for adults with dysarthria. In W. Berry (Ed.) *Clinical Dysarthria,* San Diego, California: College–Hill Press, 1983.

Hanson, W., and Metter, E. DAF as instrumental treatment for dysarthria in progressive supranuclear palsy: A case report, *Journal of Speech and Hearing Disorders,* 1980, *45*:268–276.

Hanson, W., and Metter, E. DAF speech rate modification in Parkinson's disease: A report of two cases. In W. Berry, (Ed.) *Clinical Dysarthria,* San Diego, California: College–Hill Press, 1983.

Yorkston, K. and Beukelman, D. *Assessment of Intelligibility of Dysarthric Speech.* Tigard, Oregon: C.C. Publications, 1981.

CHAPTER NINE

TREATMENT OF HYPERKINETIC DYSARTHRIA

Method of David R. Beukelman

Individuals with speech disorders secondary to excessive motor activity such as myoclonic jerks, tics, chorea, and dystonia are classified as hyperkinetic dysarthric speakers. These hyperkinesias usually result from toxic reactions to drugs, neurochemical disorders, or neurologic disorders. The severity range across hyperkinetic dysarthric speakers is extensive, with some individuals exhibiting only a trace of inconsistent impairment and others unable to communicate verbally. For example, speakers with chorea may demonstrate intelligible speech that is disrupted and distorted only at the moment of hyperkinesis. In dystonia, motor control of the speech mechanism may be gradually distorted throughout a speech utterance because of the slow dyskinesis.

The primary treatment approaches for individuals with hyperkinesis involve chemical and surgical intervention, rather than behavioral management.* The speech symptoms are so closely related to the underlying movement disorder that marked improvement in speech symptom is dependent on modification of the severity of the movement disorder.

The goals of chemical intervention efforts are to improve function, reduce destructive movement patterns, and improve cosmesis. Objective measurement of patient performance in a variety of areas is often needed to determine the overall result of adjustments in a chemical intervention program. Along with other health care professionals, I am involved in the serial measurement of patient performance. Using the *Assessment of Intelligibility of Dysarthric Speech,* speech intelligibility and speaking rate data are taken and combined into a composite measure of speech efficiency (intelligible words per minute), which is reported as a functional measure of speech performance. Sustained vowel duration, vowel and CV syllable diadochokinesis, and, at times, articulation measurements are also taken. When specific questions about respiratory support for speech, velopharyngeal port function, or phonatory quality are of concern, additional laboratory and perceptual measures are completed.

A review of the literature does not reveal research systematically documenting the effectiveness of behavioral speech treatment of hyperkinetic dysarthria. There are case studies that report favorable outcomes as the result of biofeedback treatment. My attempts at symptomatic treatment have had very limited success. Therefore, at the present time, I provide little direct speech treatment to functionally intelligible hyperkinetic dysarthric speakers.

Selected speakers receive instruction in managing verbal interaction with strangers. They are instructed to:

1. Maintain eye contact with the listener when postural position permits.

2. Inform the listener that they wish to know immediately when they have not been understood.

3. Reiterate an utterance or word when an abnormal movement pattern has potentially interfered with communication.

4. Carefully introduce the topic of discussion rather than jump from one topic to another.

For the hyperkinetic speaker who does not achieve functionally intelligible speech after chemical or surgical treatment has been used, communication-augmentative or communication-assistive approaches may be implemented. Three of my dystonic clients with adequate hand control have augmented their speech intelligibility by pointing to the first letter of each word on an alphabet board as they speak. With this additional information, listeners were able to understand the dystonic speakers. At times of communication breakdown, the entire word in question was spelled using the alphabet board. One unintelligible dystonic individual employed a scanning communication-augmentation system that was selected and customized so that health and self-care instructions were retrieved in their entirety and unique messages were spelled letter by letter.

SELECTED REFERENCES

Beukelman, D. and Yorkston, K. A communication system for the severely dysarthric speaker with an intact language system. *Journal of Speech and Hearing Disorders,* 1977, *42*:265–270.

Darley, F., Aronson, A., and Brown, J., *Motor Speech Disorders*. Philadelphia: W.B. Saunders Company, 1975.

Helme, R., Movement Disorders. In M. Samuels (Ed.), *Manual of Neurologic Therapeutics*. Boston: Little, Brown and Company, 1978.

Vinken, P., and Bruyn, G. *Handbook of Clinical Neurology* (6): *Diseases of Basal Ganglia*. New York: American Elsevier Publishing Company, Inc., 1968.

Yorkston, K. and Beukelman, D. *Assessment of Intelligibility of Dysarthric Speech,* Tigard, Oregon: CC Publications, 1981.

Ojemann, G., and Ward, A. *Abnormal Movement Disorders.* In J. Youmans (Ed.), *Neurological Surgery.* (2nd ed.) Philadelphia: W.B. Saunders Co., pp. 3821–3857, 1982.

Acknowledgment: The preparation of this chapter was supported in part by Research Grant #G008003029 from the National Institute of Handicapped Research, Department of Education, Washington, D.C. 20202.

*The Selected Reference list contains two entries that review chemical and surgical treatment of the hyperkinesias.

CHAPTER TEN

TREATMENT OF MIXED DYSARTHRIA

Method of David R. Beukelman

Mixed dysarthria refers to a disorder of motor speech that includes a broader range of dysarthric symptoms than can be clearly classified as flaccid, spastic, ataxic, hyperkinetic, or hypokinetic dysarthria. The treatment approach for a specific mixed dysarthric speaker is dependent on analysis of evaluation results. However, I will discuss general approaches to treating the mixed dysarthria of individuals who are improving as well as those with progressive diseases or syndromes.

TREATING THE IMPROVING MIXED DYSARTHRIC SPEAKER

Augmentative Approaches

During the initial stage of treatment for the improving dysarthria secondary to brain trauma, anoxia, or encephalitis, I attempt to develop some form of communication-augmentation approach to serve communication needs until functional speech has been re-established. In this case communication augmentation refers to both technical and non-technical approaches, such as signing words/letter boards, as well as electronic equipment. Assuming that the dysarthric individual's linguistic and cognitive abilities are grossly intact, selection of a communication-augmentation approach depends primarily on the individual's communication need along with the levels of motor and sensory abilities.

For severely dysarthric individuals, the length of transition period between use of communication-augmentation systems and functional speech may be considerable. In an effort to encourage development of functional speech, the dysarthric speaker may be instructed to supplement initial speech attempts with a communication aid. For example, I often instruct the speaker to point to the first letter of a word on an alphabet board as the word is spoken. This technique **105** appears to improve the intelligibility of communication exchange between speaker and listener in two ways. First, the listener is provided with additional information in the form of the first letter of the word being spoken. With this information, the listener is often able to guess the word that the speaker is producing. Second, some speakers improve intelligibility of their speech when they use this system even though the listener cannot see the alphabet board. Because their speech supplemented by the alphabet board serves a communication purpose, they tend to speak earlier in their recovery and thus increase practice time. Availability of the alphabet board during communication exchanges also provides speaker and listener with an additional means of resolving communication breakdown, as unintelligible words can be spelled using the alphabet board.

Establishing Functionally Intelligible Speech

Coordination Disorders. The treatment approaches selected to develop intelligible speech by severely dysarthric speakers depend on the pattern of motor impairment demonstrated by each client. If the predominant motor pattern involves incoordination, intelligible speech can often be achieved by reducing the rate and, thus, complexity of the motor task. When the speaking rate is decreased, the speaker is given additional time to achieve the precise articulatory targets required for intelligible speech. Furthermore, improved coordination of respiratory activity with other speech mechanism subsystems allows phonatory and articulatory behaviors to be completed in the presence of a consistent and an adequate air pressure supply. Individuals with cognitive impairment in addition to their dysarthria must often be taught to adjust speaking rate, because this type of speaker frequently does not voluntarily reduce rate to achieve intelligible speech. Depending on the learning ability of the dysarthric speaker and on the desired rate patterns, a variety of techniques for controlling rate are used.

Appropriate Pausing. Dysarthric speakers with coordination disorders frequently benefit from pausing appropriately during speech. The well-placed pause will help segment phrases of the utterance. During the pause the speech mechanism may come briefly to a nearly neutral posture or assume a "ready" posture prior to a difficult sound sequence. The influence of articulatory breakdown which may have occurred during a difficult sequence is less likely to carry over and affect the precision of subsequent sounds and words if the pause is interjected after the articulatory breakdown. Introduction of appropriately placed pauses will reduce overall speaking rate; however, rate of articulatory movement per se may or may not be reduced.

Rigid Imposition of Rate. Some individuals are able to modify speaking rate only under rigid control. This can be achieved by instructing the patient to point to the first letter of each word on an alphabet board as the word is spoken, or by training the speaker to point to successive locations on a pacing board as each word is produced. I use this technique only when others fail since it tends to encourage bizarre prosody.

Rhythmic Cueing The speaker is instructed to say each word of a message at the same time, or slightly after, the clinician has cued him by pointing to specific words in reading material. This technique controls speaking rate, but maintains some of the durational aspects of normal speech, e.g., (1) shortening the duration of primarily stressed words, and (2) pausing before and/or after phrases. I use it when the patient cannot voluntarily control speaking rate, but does not require rigid control.

Verbal Instruction. A limited number of individuals are able to modify their speaking rate consistently, following instructions to reduce rate by a given percentage. This technique allows the speaker to reduce rate according to his own strategies and does not encourage bizarreness. Speakers who are successful with this technique are usually cognitively alert and very motivated to control their speaking rate.

Throughout rate control programs, the relationship between speaking rate and speech intelligibility is closely monitored. The treatment goal is to stabilize rate so that an intelligibility level is at, or above, 90 per cent. An elevated rate results in reduced intelligibility, whereas an excessively lower rate does little to enhance intelligibility, reduces the speaker's efficiency (intelligible words per minute), and increases bizarreness. I use the *Assessment of Intelligibility of Dysarthric Speech* to measure single-word, as well as sentence, intelligibility. Speaking rate data can be collected from the same sentence samples that were used to measure intelligibility.

Strength and Speed Disorders. In cases where intelligibility is reduced primarily because of strength and speed problems, control of speaking rate will probably be a less valuable strategy to increase intelligibility than in cases with a coordination disorder. The primary treatment strategy to increase intelligibility of dysarthric individuals with speed and strength problems involves development of muscle control of the components of the speech mechanism needed to generate and valve the air pressure levels present during speech. Briefly, respiratory goals include development of rapid inhalation and extended exhalation patterns associated with normal speech. These patterns are developed first on the nonspeaking blowing tasks, and then on sustained vowel production, and finally in connection with speech. Steady control of subglottal air pressure during nonspeech tasks (Netsell and Daniel, 1979), during sustained vowels, and finally during connected speech are also necessary. Air pressure levels generated by the respiratory system during speech may be augmented by the use of abdominal binders.

The phonatory goals include ability to initiate and terminate phonation. Training to achieve this goal usually involves a variety of vowel sounds, which are sustained for varying lengths up to 5 to 10 seconds. This activity often is monitored using the intensity trace from a Visipitch unit (contact neck microphone). A second phonatory goal is initiation of phonation at the beginning of the exhalation phase of respiration. This goal was stressed early in phonatory training, during production of extended vowels, and later in connected speech activities. A third phonatory goal necessary for some speakers is to interrupt phonation several times during a single breath. This is an important prerequisite skill for appropriate pausing to signal stress and improve articulation during connected speech.

Depending on the individual speech patterns of the mixed dysarthric speaker, a variety of articulation goals are selected to increase speech intelligibility. Initially, a repertoire of three to six vowels are differentiated. This is usually achieved during early activities of phonatory/respiratory training. Approximation of stop consonants, usually bilabial and lingual alveolar, are differentiated as the first consonant sounds. Early developing consonants and vowels are combined to form functional words in both CV and VC combinations. As additional vowels and consonants are differentiated, training activities are frequently structured in a contrasted format. In this way, the speaker focuses on maximizing the intelligibility of each word so that it can be distinguished from a contrasted word.

When patients do not improve velopharyngeal closure as speaking rate is controlled, and when velopharyngeal incompetence patterns remain consistent, palatal lifts are constructed for many of our dysarthric speakers. Often the palatal lift is fitted early in treatment, so that intraoral air pressure can be successfully impounded and articulation precision can be improved during the articulation training phase of the program. Increased efficiency of the speech mechanism resulting from a velopharyngeally competent port reduces respiratory demands during speech.

Typically, dysarthric speakers cannot be involved in speech treatment for numerous hours every day, yet it is difficult for them to maximize their performance without extensive practice. For this reason, family members and other support persons are encouraged to observe treatment sessions and to play an active role in practice sessions with the speaker. Tasks are included in practice sessions only if they have been demonstrated successfully in treatment sessions. Frequently, the goal of practice is to increase reliability and accuracy of task performance, rather than to establish new movements or sequence of movements. Attempting to speak intelligibly is a very motivating method of practice. For this reason, the communication situation frequently is structured so that the speaker is encouraged early to become a functional speaker, even though his repertoire of words may be limited in the initial aspects of the program. This structuring may include the continued use of the alphabet board so that the first letter of each word can be identified as the word is spoken. Also, the words the speaker can produce are included on a master list, which is provided to staff and support persons. Knowledge of the words on the master list allows listeners to guess from a closed rather than an open set of words.

Beyond Intelligibility

Maximizing Communication Efficiency   In a narrow sense, communication efficiency can be considered as some combination of speech intelligibility and speaking rate. While maximizing communication efficiency, the maintenance of a high level of speech intelligibility (at least 90 per cent) is basic to successful communication. Once cognitively alert dysarthric speakers, other than the hypokinetic type, achieve an intelligibility level of approximately 90 per cent, they frequently are reluctant to attempt to speak at rates that will noticeably interfere with that level of intelligibility. In fact, they frequently indicate that they cannot speak any more rapidly. Often, these speakers are correct in their perceptions and are helpful in participating in the decision to determine the optimal relationship between intelligibility and speaking rate. For the less cognitively alert, considerable clinician assistance may be needed to select the optimal combination of intelligibility and rate that is effective, and then to train them to maintain these levels.

The aspect of the training program designed to increase communication efficiency usually involves use of very familiar materials, which are practiced over and over again. Tape recordings of the speaker's efforts, and subsequent evaluation of the degree to which intelligibility and precision have been maintained, are useful in assisting the patient to monitor his performance with increasing accuracy. Extensive practice periods are helpful in this phase. Usually, a supportive friend or family member should be trained to act as a supervisor of these activities, to monitor practice time, and to resolve confusion that the dysarthric speaker may have about practice assignments.

Minimizing Bizarreness. The experienced dysarthria clinician is aware that reduction of bizarreness is involved in most activities designed to increase speech intelligibility and to increase communication efficiency. Throughout the treatment program, tasks that increase bizarreness should be avoided when other tasks can be used to achieve intelligibility treatment goals. The goal of minimizing bizarreness is accomplished by achieving an appropriate speech loudness level and developing the skills necessary to signal stress appropriately.

Prosodic adjustments used to signal stress in English involve changes in pitch, loudness, and durational parameters that normal speakers shift so subtly that listeners are largely unaware of the techniques employed to signal stress. For the dysarthric speaker, control of these stressing parameters, simultaneous with production of segmental aspects of speech, requires considerable attention, and may contribute to bizarreness of the speech pattern. This bizarreness may result from (1) inadequate stressing, in which speech is judged to have a nonstressed quality, (2) stressing most words equally so that the speech is judged to have an excess and equal stress quality.

I instruct dysarthric patients to focus initially on a single parameter to signal stress. Duration usually is selected because it is a parameter that is often more easily controlled by the dysarthric speaker than intensity or pitch. Also, excess in durational adjustment is not perceived as being as bizarre as excessive loudness and pitch adjustments. In addition, adjustments in duration are frequently accompanied by subtle adjustments in loudness, which encourage natural stressing patterns. Pitch adjustments usually are reserved to signal the interrogative. Initially, adjustments in duration are trained on an imitative basis or by displaying the acoustic signal on the screen of an oscilloscope for feedback purposes. Next, contrastive stress drills are employed. The speaker is instructed to say a given sentence in response to a variety of antecedent comments or questions produced by the clinician. The speaker attempts to respond with an appropriate stressing pattern. During these activities the speaker is also told which words to avoid stressing. Often, during initial attempts to achieve stress, the dysarthric speaker will stress all words with a few words "hyperstressed." The initial target words to be unstressed are usually the articles (a, an, the), because they are typically un-stressed in English. Exceptions are learned later. Following the contrast drills, these same sentences are included in paragraph context. The speaker analyzes the content of the paragraph and attempts to use appropriate stressing patterns. Later conversational exchanges are audiotaped and reviewed to analyze appropriateness of stress patterns employed by the speaker.

TREATMENT OF THE INDIVIDUAL WITH PROGRESSIVE MIXED DYSARTHRIA

The sequencing of treatment for the individual with progressive dysarthria is quite different from that of the individual with improving dysarthria. However, many of the goals and strategies are similar. Generally, my approach to treating progressive dysarthrics can be divided into four areas—maximizing speech efficiency, maximizing intelligibility, listener training, and communication augmentation.

Maximizing Speech Efficiency. The effort required to speak extensively is often tiring to the individual with progressive neurogenic disease. One treatment goal is to minimize speaking effort and still maintain intelligible speech. Portable voice amplifiers with boom microphones attached to glasses or mounted on an ear clip are used to compensate for reduced loudness. Palatal lifts are fitted for individuals who are allowing considerable air escape through the incompetent velopharyngeal port. Depending on the degree of respiratory weakness and intension tremor, postural adjustments often reduce speech effort and increase speech efficiency. Some patients produce phonation more easily while supine than while sitting. Abdominal binders provide additional expiratory force, but the speaker must have the strength to "override" the binder on the inhalation phase of respiration. Close cooperation with a physician is needed to ensure adequate ventilation of the individual with the abdominal binder. Family members and care personnel must be instructed in binder placement to achieve desired effect and prevent secondary problems, such as inadequate ventilation of skin with consequent breakdown.

Maximizing Intelligibility. I employ several strategies to maximize and maintain the speech intelligibility of the speaker with progressive dysarthria. First, individuals with progressive dysarthria who are cognitively alert frequently adjust their speaking rate in an effort to maintain intelligible speech. However, if such adjustments are not voluntarily made, rate control training is necessary. Second, influence of omission of critical consonant sounds on intelligibility is discussed with the dysarthric individuals, and they are instructed to expend the effort necessary to produce these consonants. Third, when speech begins to require excessive effort, speakers often resort to one-word utterances or severely telegraphic speech. In an attempt to determine the influence of these speaking patterns, speech intelligibility measures—both sentence and single-word intelligibility—are taken. For moderately dysarthric speakers, speech in context is often more intelligible than single word utterances or highly telegraphic speech. For the severely dysarthric speaker, single-word intelligibility may be higher than sentence intelligibility, or there may be little difference. Fourth, dysarthric speakers are instructed to inform their listener of the topic of the conversation at the outset. This technique often prevents communication breakdown and saves communication time and effort. Fifth, the speaker is instructed to point to the first letter of each word on an alphabet board as it is spoken, spelling the entire word on the alphabet board, to efficiently resolve communication breakdown with minimal effort. This technique also is beneficial in maintaining intelligible speech.

Listener Training. Provision of information intended to prevent or resolve communication breakdown encourages more efficient communication and more harmonious interpersonal relationships. When the dysarthric individual's speech patterns show impairment in intelligibility, primary listeners are encouraged to participate in a training session. The objectives of this session are as follows:

1. Hearing acuity of each of the listeners is confirmed and those with impairment are encouraged to maximize their hearing ability through medical and audiologic care.
2. Auditory distractions in frequent communication environments are reduced or eliminated.
3. Listeners are instructed to confirm the accuracy of their understanding of what the dysarthric speaker has said, rather than attempt to guess the speaker's message.
4. Listeners are instructed to confirm the topic of the conversation with the dysarthric speaker at the beginning of the exchange.
5. Listeners receive training in the operation and management of the communication-augmentation system where appropriate.

Communication Augmentation. Communication-augmentation systems are selected for speakers with progressive dysarthria who are no longer able to produce intelligible speech. Care is taken to select systems that will serve their communication needs throughout the typical course of their disease or condition.

SELECTED REFERENCES

Beukelman, D., and Yorkston, K. A communication system for the severely dysarthric speaker with an intact language system. *Journal of Speech and Hearing Disorders* 1977, *42*:265–250.

Darley, F., Aronson, A., and Brown, M. *Motor Speech Disorders*. Philadelphia: W.B. Saunders Company, 1975.

Netsell, R., and Daniel, B. Dysarthria in adults: Physiologic approach to rehabilitation. *Archives of Physical Medicine and Rehabilitation,* 1979, *60*:502–508.

Rosenbek, J., and LaPointe, L., The dysarthrias: Description diagnosis and treatment. In D.F. Johns (Ed.), *Clinical Management of Neurogenic Communication Disorders*. Boston: Little, Brown and Company, 1978.

Yorkston, K., and Beukelman, D. *Assessment of Intelligibility of Dysarthric Speech*. Tigard, Oregon: CC Publications, 1981.

Acknowledgement: The preparation of this chapter was supported in part by Research Grant #G00803029 from the National Institute of Handicapped Research, Department of Education, Washington, D.C. 20202

CHAPTER ELEVEN

DYSARTHRIA: COMMUNICATION-AUGMENTATION SYSTEMS FOR ADULTS WITHOUT SPEECH

Method of Franklin H. Silverman

For this discussion, emphasis is on communication augmentation for the dysarthric adult who has essentially normal ability to comprehend speech and to solve problems and see relationships (i.e., function cognitively), but who lacks adequate intelligible speech to meet all of his communication needs. The prognosis for his eventually developing adequate intelligible speech could fall anywhere in the range from extremely poor to excellent. His dysarthria could have resulted from a lesion anywhere in the central or peripheral nervous system. His disturbance in motor functioning could be limited to the speech mechanism or could include one or more extremities.

Much of the information presented is applicable to communication augmentation for the cerebral-palsied child who is dysarthric. Much of it is also applicable to the dysarthric adult who has some disturbance in ability to comprehend speech or to function cognitively; the prognosis for such a person developing adequate communication to meet his needs is not as good as for one who has both normal intelligence and normal receptive-language functioning.

Intelligible speech is superior to any augmentation system as a communication medium. Hence, an effort should be made to improve muscle functioning to a level that is adequate to support increased speech intelligibility, if there is a reasonable chance of being successful. Communication augmentation should *not* be delayed, however, until an attempt has been made to develop intelligible speech. There has been much research that indicates that intervention with an augmentative communication system not only does not interfere with the development of intelligible speech in severely communicatively handicapped persons, but, in approximately one-third of the cases, appears to facilitate it. Also, even if the prognosis for developing

115

intelligible speech is excellent, a dysarthric is quite likely to benefit from being interfaced with a communication-augmentation system until his speech becomes adequate to meet his communication needs.

GENERAL PRINCIPLES OF INTERVENTION WITH COMMUNICATION AUGMENTATIVES

Rehabilitating an adult dysarthric, utilizing one or more communication-augmentation systems, involves (1) identifying the *optimal* system (or combination of systems) for meeting his communication needs, (2) interfacing him with the system (or systems) identified, and (3) periodically reassessing the ability of the system (or systems) selected to continue meeting his communication needs.

The first task is identifying the *optimal* augmentation system (or combination of systems) for the client. This is the system (or systems) that, when combined with his existing communication abilities, comes closest to meeting his communication needs efficiently. To identify this system (or systems), I first attempt to establish which of the available augmentation systems the client has the motor, sensory, and cognitive abilities to use (Silverman, 1980). After I have identified this subset of systems, I then decide which of them (or which combination of them) appears to be optimal for meeting the client's communication needs. When making this decision, I consider such factors as the extent to which each possible system (or combination) would allow the person to meet his communication needs, the cost of the hardware and software components for each possible system (or combination), the length of time it would take the client to learn to use each possible system (or combination), the extent to which using each is likely to interfere with the client's ongoing activity, the intelligibility of the messages communicated by each to untrained observers, and the acceptability of each to users and interpreters.

After I have identified what appears to be the optimal system (or systems) for the client, my next task is to interface him with it (or them). This ordinarily involves the acquisition (for systems with electronic displays) or construction (for nonelectronic communication boards) of the "hardware" components of the system and the selection of "software" components—i.e., message components, or symbols, to be included on, or generated by, the display (e.g., words, letters of the alphabet, photographs, Blissymbols, or Rebus symbols). If a dysarthric adult had sufficiently good control of at least one upper extremity for a gestural system (such as Amer-Ind) to be optimal, there would be no need to acquire or construct hardware components; there would, of course, still be a need to select software components— i.e., the specific signs to be taught.

After I have selected the software components for the system and have acquired or constructed any hardware components that are necessary for implementing it, I am ready to teach the client to use the system. The length of time this takes is a function of both the amount he has to learn before he will be capable of using the system and his learning ability. The *less* the client has to learn and the *better* his learning ability, the *shorter* the time period that ordinarily is required before he is capable of using it for communicating. If the client is familiar with the message components (e.g., words) being used and is able to make the muscle gestures, or movements, required for activating the switching mechanism or for indicating message components on the display (if a communication board is used), the amount of time required for teaching him to use the system can be less than one hour.

A communication-augmentation system that is optional at the time of the initial assessment for meeting the client's communication needs may not remain optimal over time. His communication needs are likely to change: as his rehabilitation program progresses and as he is expected to interact with more persons in more environments, both his vocabulary needs and his message transmission needs are likely to change. The vocabulary set that was adequate for communicating in the hospital or nursing home may be inadequate for communicating in the home or office. Also, if he improves sufficiently to be able to return to his job, he may require an augmentation system capable of transmitting written and telephone messages as well as face-to-face ones.

Another reason why a client's communication system(s) may not remain optimal over time is that his motor, sensory, and/or cognitive status may change. If the neurological condition that caused the dysarthria is a progressive one (such as ALS), the client's motor, sensory, and/or cognitive abilities are likely to deteriorate. Such deterioration could impede his ability to use the system(s) with which he was initially interfaced.

Since there is a high probability that an adult dysarthric's communication-augmentation system(s) will not remain optimal over time, there is a need for periodic reassessment, perhaps as often as every 2 or 3 months. The interval between reassessments for a given client would be determined by several factors, including the rate at which his motor, sensory, and cognitive status was changing and the rate at which his communication needs were changing.

SOME SPECIFIC CONSIDERATIONS AND SUGGESTIONS RELEVANT TO DESIGNING COMMUNICATION-AUGMENTATION SYSTEMS FOR DYSARTHRIC ADULTS

There are a number of factors that I consider when interfacing a dysarthric adult with a communication-augmentation system. For in-depth considerations of these factors, see Chapters 5 through 8 in *Communication for the Speechless* (Silverman, 1980). Some of the more important are:

1. *Choice of System: Electronic versus Nonelectronic.* Almost any dysarthric adult who can be interfaced with an electronic communication augmentation system can also be interfaced with a nonelectronic system, or communication board. Although an electronic system may permit a dysarthric to communicate at a faster rate, and in more situations than would a communication board, electronic systems tend to be more expensive, less portable, and less reliable than communication boards. Hence, it is desirable to interface all dysarthric adults, including those who will be (or have been) interfaced with an electronic communication system, with a communication board that will allow for at least basic-need communication. Such a device can serve a dysarthric as a communication medium when his electronic system is not available.

Information about commercially available communication-augmentation systems and components for such systems can be found in the *Non-Vocal Communication Resource Book* (Vanderheiden, 1978). Periodic supplements to the material presented in this loose-leaf book are issued by the Trace Research and Development Center for the Severely Communicatively Handicapped, University of Wisconsin-Madison.

2. *Choice of Indicating Mode: Direct-Selection versus Scanning versus Encoding.* Regardless of whether a dysarthric is interfaced with a communication board or an electronic system, his clinician has to decide how he will indicate the message components that he wishes to transmit. There are *three basic strategies* that he can use for this purpose: direct-selection, scanning, or encoding.

The most efficient of the three strategies is *direct-selection.* A client who is using this strategy directly selects the message components he wishes to transmit. If he is using a communication board, he indicates the message components that he wishes to transmit on it by pointing to them with a finger or a headstick or by directing his gaze at them. Or if he is using an electronic system, he uses a switching mechanism (usually containing more than one switch) to cause the display to indicate directly the message components that he wishes to transmit. To be able to use this strategy, a client must be sufficiently intact motorically to make a gesture (or series of gestures) that would allow him to point to message components on a communication board, or to activate a switching mechanism containing *more than one* switch.

If a client can somehow signal "yes" and "no," or can activate a switching mechanism containing a single switch, he can use a *scanning* strategy to indicate message components. A client who is using this strategy to indicate message components on a communication board signals "yes" or "no" as the person with whom he is attempting to communicate points to each of the various message components on his board. A client who is using this strategy to indicate message components on an electronic display activates a switch to stop the scan when a desired message component is indicated (e.g., when a rotating pointer points to the message component that he wishes to transmit). Almost any client who can be interfaced with an electronic augmentation system by using a scanning response mode can be interfaced with a communication board by using a scanning response mode.

The third indicating strategy—*encoding*—is a variation of direct-selection. The client, rather than transmitting message components directly, transmits a code (one or more symbols), which the "listener" decodes. He can use either a communication board or an electronic display to transmit the code. By selecting any two of the first seven digits, for example, he can transmit any one of 49 message components; the first digit can indicate the row, and the second the column, in a seven-row, seventeen-column (49-cell) square matrix in which each cell contains a message component.

3. *Choice of Symbol Set.* If a client's reading and spelling abilities are within normal limits, I ordinarily choose a symbol set consisting of the letters of the alphabet and some words and phrases that he is apt to use a great deal. With this symbol set he could transmit any message. If his reading ability is fairly good, but his spelling ability is poor, I ordinarily choose a symbol set consisting of words and phrases. Such a symbol set obviously would only allow him to communicate a limited number of messages—preferably those that it would be important for him to be able to transmit. If both his reading and spelling abilities are poor, I ordinarily would choose a symbol set consisting of photographs and/or drawings. This type of symbol set, like the previous one, allows only a limited number of messages to be transmitted. Because photographs and drawings tend to take up more space on a display than do words and phrases, fewer of them can be placed on a display. Hence, a symbol set consisting

of photographs and/or drawings usually allows a client to communicate fewer messages than a symbol set consisting of words and phrases.

If an adult dysarthric who is severely impaired motorically appears to have good spelling ability, I may consider using a symbol set consisting of the International Morse Code dot-dash signals for the letters of the alphabet. There are several ways by which he might be able to signal dots and dashes. If he can independently blink his eyes, blinking his left eye could signal a dot, and blinking his right eye a dash. Or, if he can direct his gaze in two directions, directing it in one direction can be used to signal a dot, and in the other, a dash. Or, if he can activate a two-switch switching mechanism (e.g., two myoswitches that are activated by muscle action potentials), he can input dot-dash configurations into a small computer, which can be programmed to translate the code configurations into letters of the alphabet and print them on the screen of a CRT (television) display.

Further information about selecting symbol sets for adult dysarthrics is presented in Chapters 5 and 6 of *Communication for the Speechless.*

THE POTENTIAL OF REHABILITATION WITH COMMUNICATION AUGMENTATIVES

I have outlined an approach in this paper that can be used for rehabilitating adults who are severely communicatively handicapped because of dysarthria. One may very legitimately ask whether the necessary expenditure of time and money is justified by the results. The data that have been reported on the impacts of intervention with communication augmentatives on the abilities of adult dysarthrics to communicate (e.g., Silverman, 1980, Chapters 1 and 2) suggest that such intervention can improve the communication ability of almost any adult dysarthric for whom speech alone is inadequate to meet communication needs. The degree to which a particular dysarthric would be likely to benefit would be a function of several factors including motivation to communicate, degree of motor impairment in the extremities (particularly the upper extremities) and the head and neck, degree of disturbance in the ability to comprehend speech, degree of disturbance in the ability to solve problems and see relationships, and degree of disturbance in sensory functioning. For most adult dysarthrics, the necessary expenditure of time and money is small considering the result—the ability to interact with persons, a necessary ability for truly human functioning.

SELECTED REFERENCES

Silverman, F., *Communication for the Speechless*. Englewood Cliffs, New Jersey: Prentice Hall, 1980.

Skelly, M. *Amer-Ind Gestural Code*. New York: Elsevier, 1979.

Vanderheiden, G. (Ed.). *Non-Vocal Communication Resource Book*. Baltimore: University Park Press, 1978.

INDEX